Holistic and Complementary Therapies

Updated 1st Edition

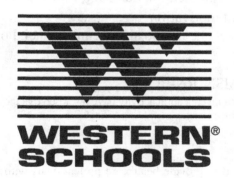

WESTERN® SCHOOLS

By
**Mercy Mammah Popoola,
RN, PhD, CNS, FWACN**

Upon successful completion of this course, continuing education hours will be awarded as follows:

Nurses: 15 Contact Hours*

*Western Schools is accredited as a provider of continuing nursing education by the American Nurses Credentialing Center's Commission on Accreditation.

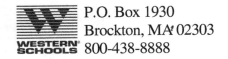
P.O. Box 1930
Brockton, MA 02303
800-438-8888

ABOUT THE AUTHOR

Mercy Mammah Popoola, RN, PhD, CNS, FWACN, is a holistic nurse and associate professor at Clayton College and State University, School of Nursing, Morrow, GA. She teaches pharmacology; nonpharmacological therapeutic modalities; natural, alternative, and complementary therapies; holistic wound healing, and the international study and internship programs. She is an active member of the American Holistic Nurses Association. Dr. Popoola received her diploma in nursing from the Eku Baptist Medical Center and School of Nursing in Eku, Nigeria, where she taught nursing for 4 years with a holistic philosophy before coming to the United States. She received her BSN at Mississippi College, Clinton, MS; her MSN at the University of Mississippi Medical Center, School of Nursing, Jackson, MS; and her PhD at the University of Colorado Health Science Center, School of Nursing, Denver, CO. She has developed many educational programs across the country. She is a wellness consultant and a Fellow of the West African College of Nursing (FWACN).

Dr. Popoola has disclosed that she has no significant financial or other conflicts of interest pertaining to this course book.

ABOUT THE CONTENT EDITOR

Yvonne Smith, MS, RN, CNS, is an undergraduate program coordinator at the University of Adron College of Nursing. In this role, Ms. Smith has leadership, management, and teaching responsibilities in a large baccalaureate program. As a health and wellness consultant, Ms. Smith has given numerous presentations and has authored several publications on such topics as complementary therapies, nutrition, health and wellness, leadership, and motivation.

Yvonne Smith has disclosed that she has no significant financial or other conflicts of interest pertaining to this course book.

Nurse Planner: Kim V. Cheramie, MSN, RN-BC

The planners who worked on this continuing education activity have disclosed that they have no significant financial or other conflicts of interest pertaining to this course book.

Copy Editor: Jamie Stockslager Boss

Indexer: Judi Gibbs

Western Schools' courses are designed to provide healthcare professionals with the educational information they need to enhance their career development as well as to work collaboratively on improving patient care. The information provided within these course materials is the result of research and consultation with prominent healthcare authorities and is, to the best of our knowledge, current and accurate at the time of printing. However, course materials are provided with the understanding that Western Schools is not engaged in offering legal, medical, or other professional advice.

Western Schools' courses and course materials are not meant to act as a substitute for seeking professional advice or conducting individual research. When the information provided in course materials is applied to individual cases, all recommendations must be considered in light of each case's unique circumstances.

Western Schools' course materials are intended solely for your use and not for the purpose of providing advice or recommendations to third parties. Western Schools absolves itself of any responsibility for adverse consequences resulting from the failure to seek medical, or other professional advice. Western Schools further absolves itself of any responsibility for updating or revising any programs or publications presented, published, distributed, or sponsored by Western Schools unless otherwise agreed to as part of an individual purchase contract.

Products (including brand names) mentioned or pictured in Western Schools' courses are not endorsed by Western Schools, any of its accrediting organizations, or any state licensing board.

ISBN: 978-1-68041-013-6

COURSE INSTRUCTIONS
IMPORTANT: Read these instructions *BEFORE* proceeding!

HOW TO EARN CONTINUING EDUCATION HOURS

To earn continuing education hour(s) and receive a certificate of completion, you must read the entire course, pass the final exam with a score of 75% or higher, and complete the course evaluation. **Unless otherwise indicated, continuing education hours will be awarded for up to 1 year from the date on which this course was purchased.**

FINAL EXAM

Enclosed with your course book you will find a FasTrax answer sheet and a FasTrax instruction sheet. Use the answer sheet to answer all of the final exam questions that appear in this course. FasTrax answer sheets are preprinted with your name and address and the course title. If you are completing more than one course, be sure to record your answers on the correct corresponding answer sheet.

Use blue or black ink to completely fill in the circles on the answer sheet. The FasTrax grading system will not read pencil. If you make an error, you may use correction fluid (such as Wite-Out®) to correct it. If the course has fewer than 100 questions, leave any remaining answer circles on the answer sheet blank.

You must score 75% or higher in order to pass this course. Should you fail to achieve the minimum required score, an additional answer sheet will be sent to you so that you may make a second attempt to pass the course. You will be allowed three attempts to pass this course. After three failed attempts, your file will be closed.

COURSE EVALUATIONS

The course evaluation provided in this course book is a required component of the course and must be completed and submitted with your final exam. Responses to evaluation statements should be recorded in the right-hand column of the answer sheet, in the section marked "Evaluation." Your evaluation provides Western Schools with vital feedback.

To provide additional feedback regarding this course, our services, or to suggest new course topics, complete the Important Information form found on the back of the instruction sheet. Return this completed form to Western Schools with your answer sheet.

SUBMITTING THE FINAL EXAM AND EVALUATION

The instruction sheet provides detailed steps for submitting your completed answer sheet and Important Information form. If you are mailing your answer sheet and Important Information form to Western Schools, we recommend that you keep a copy as a back-up.

CHANGE OF ADDRESS?

In the event that your postal or email address changes prior to completing this course, please contact our customer service department at 800-618-1670, or customerservice@westernschools.com, so that we may update your file.

WESTERN SCHOOLS GUARANTEES YOUR SATISFACTION

If any continuing education course fails to meet your expectations, or if you are not satisfied for any reason, you may return the course materials for an exchange or a refund (less shipping and handling) within 30 days, provided that you have not already received continuing education credit for the course. Software, video, and audio courses must be returned unopened. Textbooks must not be written in or marked up in any other way.

Thank you for using Western Schools to fulfill your continuing education needs!

WESTERN SCHOOLS
P.O. Box 1930
Brockton, MA 02303
800-438-8888
www.westernschools.com

WESTERN SCHOOLS
COURSE EVALUATION

HOLISTIC AND COMPLEMENTARY THERAPIES

INSTRUCTIONS: Using the scale below, please respond to the following evaluation statements. All responses should be recorded in the right-hand column of the FasTrax answer sheet, in the section marked "Evaluation." Be sure to fill in each corresponding answer circle completely using blue or black ink. Leave any remaining answer circles blank.

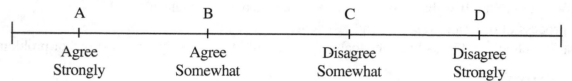

A	B	C	D
Agree Strongly	Agree Somewhat	Disagree Somewhat	Disagree Strongly

OBJECTIVES: After completing this course, I am able to:

1. Explain the history and use of the holistic philosophy, the concept of holism, and the various types of holistic, alternative, and complementary therapies.

2. Recognize and describe the various types of commonly used holistic, complementary, and alternative healing therapies.

3. Discuss the history, properties, and actions of aromatherapy and herbal therapy and relate its uses as a holistic alternative and complementary therapy.

4. Describe the history and practice of reflexology, aquatic therapy, and music therapy and relate its uses as a holistic alternative and complementary therapy.

5. Discuss the history and practice of yoga and meditation therapy and relate their uses as holistic alternative and complementary therapies.

6. Describe the history and practice of touch therapies, such as massage therapy and therapeutic touch, and relate their uses as holistic alternative and complementary therapies.

7. Describe the history and practice of folk healing and relate its uses as a holistic alternative and complementary therapy.

8. Discuss the history and practice of spiritual healing therapies, such as prayer, and relate their uses as holistic alternative and complementary therapies.

9. Discuss the practice of relaxation therapy and relate its uses as a holistic alternative and complementary therapy.

10. Discuss the history and practice of nutrition therapy and relate its uses as a holistic alternative and complementary therapy.

COURSE CONTENT

11. The course content was presented in a well-organized and clearly written manner.

12. The course content was presented in a fair, unbiased and balanced manner.

13. The course content presented current developments in the field.

14. The course was relevant to my professional practice or interests.

15. The final examination was at an appropriate level for the content of the course.

16. The course expanded my knowledge and enhanced my skills related to the subject matter.

continued on next page

17. I intend to apply the knowledge and skills I've learned to my practice.

    A. Yes   B. Unsure   C. No   D. Not Applicable

CUSTOMER SERVICE

The following section addresses your experience in interacting with Western Schools. Use the scale below to respond to the statements in this section.

    A. Yes   B. No   C. Not Applicable

18. Western Schools staff was responsive to my request for disability accommodations.
19. The Western Schools website was informative and easy to navigate.
20. The process of ordering was easy and efficient.
21. Western Schools staff was knowledgeable and helpful in addressing my questions or problems.

ATTESTATION

22. I certify that I have read the course materials and personally completed the final examination based on the material presented. Mark "A" for Agree and "B" for Disagree.

COURSE RATING

23. My overall rating for this course is

    A. Poor   B. Below Average   C. Average   D. Good   E. Excellent

You may be contacted within 3 to 6 months of completing this course to participate in a brief survey to evaluate the impact of this course on your clinical practice and patient/client outcomes.

Note: To provide additional feedback regarding this course, Western Schools services, or to suggest new course topics, use the space provided on the Important Information form found on the back of the FasTrax instruction sheet included with your course.

CONTENTS

FIGURES AND TABLES

PRETEST

1. Begin this course by taking the pretest. Circle the answers to the questions on this page, or write the answers on a separate sheet of paper. Do not log answers to the pretest questions on the FasTrax test sheet included with the course.

2. Compare your answers to the pretest key located at the end of the pretest. The pretest key indicates the chapter where the content of that question is discussed. Make note of the questions you missed, so that you can focus on those areas as you complete the course.

3. Complete the course by reading the chapters and completing the exam questions at the end of each chapter. Answers to the exam questions should be logged on the FasTrax test sheet included with the course.

Note: Choose the one option that BEST answers each question.

1. Peppermint (*Mentha piperita*) is commonly used as an
   a. antiulcer agent.
   b. antiinflammatory.
   c. antispasmodic.
   d. antidepressant.

2. Licorice (*Glycyrrhiza glabra*) is commonly used as an
   a. antiulcer agent.
   b. antidepressant.
   c. antihypertensive.
   d. antitumor agent.

3. The Zone Theory of Foot Reflexology was developed by
   a. Dr. William Fitzgerald.
   b. Dr. Joe Shelby Riley.
   c. Eunice Ingham.
   d. the Chinese.

4. Aquatic therapy can be defined as a
   a. purposeful progression of skills focusing on psychosocial and physiological functioning of water.
   b. random selection of skills focusing on psychosocial, cognitive, leisure, and motor performance using the properties of water.
   c. random selection of skills focusing on motor performance using the properties of water.
   d. purposeful progression of skills focusing on psychosocial, cognitive, leisure, and motor performance using the properties of water.

5. The recuperative and healing properties of aquatic therapy are based on
   a. hydrostatic pressure.
   b. buoyancy factor associated with water and resistance.
   c. safety factor of water and the weather factor.
   d. mechanical and thermal effects of water.

continued on next page

6. The U.S. National Association of Music Therapy was formed in

   a. 1953.
   b. 1960.
   c. 1950.
   d. 1958.

7. The holistic therapy associated with memories, fantasies, dreams, and visions is

   a. acupuncture.
   b. meditation.
   c. therapeutic touch.
   d. guided imagery.

8. Yoga is a holistic complementary therapy that is considered a type of

   a. religion.
   b. philosophy.
   c. hypnosis.
   d. acupuncture.

9. The book *Yoga Sutras* by Patanjali, which contains the eight steps of classical yoga, is mostly written in

   a. Niyama.
   b. Pranayama.
   c. Sanskrit.
   d. Dharana.

10. According to the American Institute of Holistic Theology, the seven chakras are

    a. vortices located primarily at the base of the spine.
    b. vortices located primarily at the crown of the head.
    c. bioenergetic activity radiating from bundles of energy clusters.
    d. new fibers that grow with the perfection of yoga and meditation.

11. The techniques of massage therapy, including light pressure, rubbing and kneading, pressing, vibration, tapping, and circulating pressure, originate from

    a. Swedish massage.
    b. Chinese massage.
    c. Japanese massage.
    d. African massage.

12. In classical massage, the stroking movement is referred to as

    a. vibration.
    b. effleurage.
    c. tapotement.
    d. petrissage.

13. Which statement about therapeutic touch is true?

    a. It is a specific religious practice.
    b. It is based on the philosophies of many religions.
    c. It is a cult religious practice.
    d. It is based on energy fields.

14. Dermabrasive is a folk healing practice common to

    a. Egyptians.
    b. Africans.
    c. Chinese.
    d. Caribbeans.

15. The holistic therapy in which remedies or medicines are usually manufactured from natural substances, such as plants, metals, minerals, and venoms, is

    a. Chinese medicine.
    b. aromatherapy.
    c. herbal therapy.
    d. homeopathy.

16. The act of alleged healing through the power to cause a cure or recovery from an illness or injury without the aid of conventional medical treatment is referred to as

    a. Islam.

    b. faith healing.

    c. prayer.

    d. spiritual healing practice.

17. Therapeutic Touch is a type of

    a. religious practice.

    b. philosophy.

    c. cult practice.

    d. spiritual healing practice.

18. One gram of alcohol produces

    a. 4 calories.

    b. 9 calories.

    c. 6 calories.

    d. 7 calories.

19. One gram of protein equals

    a. 6 kilocalories.

    b. 4 kilocalories.

    c. 9 kilocalories.

    d. 2 kilocalories.

20. The popular diet plan that most closely resembles a traditional diet plan and contains mostly nonprocessed foods is the

    a. Atkins diet.

    b. Mediterranean diet.

    c. vegetarian diet.

    d. Weigh Down Diet.

PRETEST KEY		
1.	C	Chapter 4
2.	A	Chapter 4
3.	C	Chapter 5
4.	D	Chapter 6
5.	D	Chapter 6
6.	C	Chapter 7
7.	D	Chapter 7
8.	B	Chapter 8
9.	C	Chapter 8
10.	C	Chapter 8
11.	B	Chapter 9
12.	B	Chapter 9
13.	D	Chapter 9
14.	B	Chapter 10
15.	D	Chapter 10
16.	B	Chapter 11
17.	D	Chapter 9 or 11
18.	D	Chapter 13
19.	B	Chapter 13
20.	B	Chapter 13

INTRODUCTION

COURSE OBJECTIVES

After completing this course, the learner will be able to:

1. Explain the history and use of the holistic philosophy, the concept of holism, and the various types of holistic, alternative, and complementary therapies.

2. Recognize and describe the various types of commonly used holistic, complementary, and alternative healing therapies.

3. Discuss the history, properties, and actions of aromatherapy and herbal therapy and relate its uses as a holistic alternative and complementary therapy.

4. Describe the history and practice of reflexology, aquatic therapy, and music therapy and relate its uses as a holistic alternative and complementary therapy.

5. Discuss the history and practice of yoga and meditation therapy and relate their uses as holistic alternative and complementary therapies.

6. Describe the history and practice of touch therapies, such as massage therapy and therapeutic touch, and relate their uses as holistic alternative and complementary therapies.

7. Describe the history and practice of folk healing and relate its uses as a holistic alternative and complementary therapy.

8. Discuss the history and practice of spiritual healing therapies, such as prayer, and relate their uses as holistic alternative and complementary therapies.

9. Discuss the practice of relaxation therapy and relate its uses as a holistic alternative and complementary therapy.

10. Discuss the history and practice of nutrition therapy and relate its uses as a holistic alternative and complementary therapy.

The revolution and reconceptualization of health and healing that has occurred in the Western health care system in the last 20 years has given opportunity for a paradigmatic shift in health care education, research, and practice. One hundred years ago, the American health care system was dominated by the biomedical worldview. Today, this is no longer true. Support for complementary and alternative medicine (CAM), also called natural, alternative, and complementary (NAC) therapies and holistic practices, has never been greater than at the present time. In a study by Eisenberg et al. (1993), 34% of the 1,539 adults surveyed reported using at least one unconventional therapy in the past year and one-third saw alternative therapy practitioners. In 1998, Eisenberg et al. again reported increased use of CAM by the American public. This recent public support for and embracement of CAM led Congress in 1994 to pass the Dietary Supplement and Health Education Act for the use of herbal remedies. It has also led to the recognition of CAM and the holistic approach to practice in the present health care system and in stress and disease management (Lilley & Aucker, 2003).

In this course book, the terms *complementary, alternative, nonconventional,* and *natural medicine and therapies* are used interchangeably. However, technically speaking, complementary therapy is used as an adjunct to conventional medicine (for example, when a patient takes a drug but also uses proper nutrition). On the other hand, alternative medicine is used in place of conventional medicine (for example, drinking the right tea or using music therapy, rather than taking a sleeping pill, to create an environment that promotes sleep). *CAM* is the term most commonly used by the National Center for Complementary and Alternative Medicine (NCCAM), medical professionals, and the majority of the public. However, *NAC therapy* is a newer term used mostly by the American Holistic Nurses Association and by nurses that include natural and traditional health care practices not included in CAM.

Stress is a real phenomenon. It is an effect of overactivity of the sympathetic nervous system that produces physical, emotional, economic, and spiritual imbalance. The issues of stress, burnout, and stress-related illness have been recognized in health care since the beginning of nursing and medical practice. Stress has been linked to or found to produce such stress-related physical illnesses as hypertension, anxiety disorders, obesity, and headaches and is a major cause of psychological illness and spiritual imbalance. In fact, stress has a holistic component in that the effects of stress can be physical, social, emotional, spiritual, economic, and even political. Possible effects of stress include angina, physical illnesses, peptic ulcers, motor vehicle and other accidents, emotional imbalance, panic attacks, depression, eating disorders, dysfunctional families, family role crises, homelessness, and isolation. Some examples of causes of stress are inability to pay bills, bankruptcy, budget crises, job stressors or politics, arrogant coworkers, political statements, riots, wars, and religious conflicts or isolation.

Stress has become a household, health care, and office word, and CAM therapies such as music therapy, herbal therapy, art, dance, exercise, relaxation exercises, yoga, meditation, aromatherapy, and humor therapy are among the healing and relaxation activities that are often used to cope with life stressors. Many health care providers and the public have come to realize that these therapeutics hold the potential to achieve balance and healing of the body, mind, and spirit.

The concept of energy in healing and its use as a philosophy for promoting holistic healing is not new. Energy healing has been used for generations in numerous health care settings to achieve various therapeutic effects, for example, to promote sleep, reduce anxiety, and treat illnesses. Energy therapies are ancient healing practices grounded in the premise that the body, mind, spirit, and emotions form a complex dynamic energy field that can be manipulated to promote holistic healing.

Also known as *biofield therapies,* energy therapies are not only approved by the NCCAM but are also endorsed by the American Nurses Association. Touch therapy is one type of energy therapy that is used to stimulate the energy channels of the body to help restore balance or maintain homeostasis. Shiatzu is another form of touch therapy in which a practitioner uses the thumbs or heel of the hand for deep pressure massage along energy lines. Another touch therapy called *effleurage* is commonly used during labor and delivery to help in the management of pain.

To understand how the universe impacts healing, practitioners must be open to understanding the major paradigm shift that has occurred across the sciences – from physics to medicine – over the centuries. Science used to rely heavily or solely on a mechanistic Newtonian model of the universe that viewed the world as a great machine. Under this thinking, humans were reduced and compartmentalized like machines. Today, however, science is exploring other paradigms of knowing. One such change in thinking includes a model based on the Einsteinian paradigm of a complex, yet interconnected, energetic-field-like universe (Breiner, 1993). This new science is interested in the whole process and sees the whole person as interconnected, with room for creativity, consciousness raising, and reciprocal interaction and tendencies. It is also dynamic and relational with humans. In Einstein's new paradigm, all matter – including the human body – is a manifestation of energy. Under this new paradigm, which is based on the beliefs of many ancient cultures, illness and stress are viewed as interruptions in the flow of energy in our bodies. The goal, therefore, in healing and promoting wholeness (holism) is to attempt to rebalance the energy flow. An understanding of the energy therapeutics and other types of CAM that will be discussed in this book can help us to better appreciate the human potential for self-healing and the concept of holism in healing.

Holism is defined as a philosophy that views everything in terms of patterns of organization, relationships, interactions, and processes that combine to form a whole. Massage, aromatherapy, yoga, exercise, reflexology, meditation, Therapeutic Touch, guided imagery, and herb, music, aquatic, and nutrition therapy are some holistic modalities that have been found to be useful in the treatment of certain ailments, in stress reduction, and in healing. Historically, however, healing has been viewed in diverse ways (Anumolu, Miller, Popoola, Talley, & Rushing, 2004; Dossey, 2001). The majority of the time, our viewpoints are shaped by our worldviews (biomedical or holistic). The ultimate goal of CAM, however, is not simply to promote healing but to induce or maintain a state of balance, harmony, and wholeness (body, mind, and spirit). Therefore, an understanding of the concepts of energy and holism are critical to the understanding of the holistic healing process and the management of stress-related diseases. Nightingale, in 1859, and Dossey, in 2001, emphasized this point when they noted that healing is not synonymous with curing, but that healing comes with the process of creating and promoting a holistic environment. The best way to present the difference between healing and curing, therefore, is to revisit the concept of healing from a holistic perspective, using the evolution of CAM or NAC therapies in the last two decades.

This course is designed for nurses and other health care providers to facilitate and inspire experience with alternative and complementary therapeutic modalities while appreciating the role of holism in healing and stress management. The goal is to promote the use and praxis of different types of holistic NAC therapies for healing, stress, and disease management.

CHAPTER 1

THE HOLISTIC PHILOSOPHY

CHAPTER OBJECTIVE

Upon completion of this chapter, the learner will be able to explain the history and use of the holistic philosophy, the concept of holism, and the various types of holistic, alternative, and complementary therapies.

LEARNING OBJECTIVES

After studying this chapter, the learner will be able to:

1. Discuss the history of complementary and alternative therapies.
2. Explain the concept of holism and its application in healing.
3. Identify the most commonly used complementary and alternative therapies in healing.
4. Differentiate the different types of complementary and alternative therapies appropriate to and common to different populations.

HISTORY OF COMPLEMENTARY AND ALTERNATIVE THERAPY PRACTICE

The art of healing comes from nature, not from the physician. Therefore the physician must start from nature, with an open mind.
Paracelcus, (1493-1541)

The use of complementary and alternative medicine (CAM) in healing is not new; these therapies date to the beginning of civilization. In fact, long before any scientific tools were available, and documented as far back as 1500 B.C., the Egyptians and the Chinese used herbs, massage, aromatherapy, hydrotherapy, plasters, bandages, oils, honey, and copper as treatments (Keegan, 1998). However, as society and cultures became increasingly multicultural, multisocial, and multitechnological, many traditional healing practices were renamed, changed, and reconceptualized to meet the demands and health care needs of our changing world (Popoola, 2003a).

With the incidence and prevalence of chronic and stress-related illnesses rising, even despite advances in science and technology, the need to revisit alternative and complementary therapies should be a major focus in health care and in stress management today. Health care providers who understand the traditions and alternative practices used in disease management would be able to provide a beneficial contribution towards the overall health of their patients.

TRENDS IN CAM

In the 1960s, the public expressed concerns over the iatrogenic effects of conventional medicines. Although today there is more attention given to the prevention of illness and disease, there remains frustration over a fragmented health care system, which is still highly cure- and medication-focused, and even more specialized, segmented and time-constrained than ever. Current health care practice focuses mainly on the use of drugs in disease management, although the potential and actual disease-producing side effects of drugs are well known. For example, when taken for asthma, the drug prednisone could potentially produce other diseases and complications, such as hypertension, diabetes, peptic ulcers, osteoporosis, slow wound healing, body image disturbances, mood changes, and depression. As more specialized health care providers become involved in disease-narrowed aspects of the patient, along with greater quantities of available drugs (both prescription and OTC), there is an exponentially higher risk of drug-drug interactions, allergic responses, side-effects, overdose, and sometimes fatal adverse events. This knowledge has created a renewed interest in and growing recognition of natural, alternative, and complementary (NAC) therapies.

In 1998, the National Institutes of Health (NIH) in Washington, D.C., established the National Center for Complementary and Alternative Medicine (NCCAM), a federal government agency devoted to rigorous evidence-based research on health care systems, practices, and products that are beyond the scope of conventional medicine. NCCAM's mission is to provide information on the safety and efficacy of complementary and alternative therapies, ensuring that health care professionals and the public have the most current and comprehensive data regarding use and integration of these approaches (NCCAM, 2014a).

THE HOLISTIC APPROACH

What Is Holism?

The root of the word "holism" is the Greek *holos*, which means "whole." Central to the philosophy and practice of complementary and alternative medicine (CAM) is the concept of holism,

which is the belief of caring for the whole person – body, mind and spirit – and not just the illness, with a goal of reaching optimal health and wellness. The holistic and biomedical healing approaches operate from two separate paradigms. Biomedical approaches are mechanistic and objective, with a focus on curing. Holistic approaches are dynamic and interactive, with a focus on healing based on a philosophy of care (Popoola, 2000a; Popoola, 2003b). Table 1-1 presents the differences between the holistic and biomedical approaches to healing.

Caring for clients from the holistic perspective has been the unique function of nurses since the time of Florence Nightingale. Although holism is central to the nursing profession, the concept of holism, unlike other nursing concepts such as caring, self-care, and energy fields, has not been fully developed and operationally defined.

Philosophy

The concept of holism was first introduced in 1926 by South African statesman and biologist Jan Christian Smuts, who presented living things as more than the sum of their parts. Unlike modern approaches that dehumanize clients, this holistic approach is humanistic and considers the environment, the culture, and the interconnection between humans and the other forms of life and energy on Earth.

Einstein is among the many great intellectuals who helped to move conventional science from the mechanistic Newtonian perspective to an understanding that all matter on earth and within the universe is energetically connected as a whole. In Einstein's famous equation ($E=mc^2$), he noted that all matter is a manifestation of energy. Paradoxically, this formula and its concept of energy were the bases for the formation of the atomic bomb. According to Einstein, all forms of mass, including the human

TABLE 1-1: DIFFERENCES BETWEEN THE BIOMEDICAL AND HOLISTIC APPROACHES TO HEALING		
Concept	**Biomedical Approach**	**Holistic Approach**
Worldview	Positivistic and mechanistic	Humanistic and holistic
Mind	Separate from the body	Mind and body, same process
Nature of knowledge	From the context	In context
Goal	Empirical control	Wisdom and many views
View of Human	Objective	Subjective
Drive or value	Technological or machine	Human value
Care and treatment	Fragmented	Dynamic and interactive
Treatment focus	Curing	Healing
Outcome	Measurable and mathematical	Holism and balance
Financial effect	Costly and materialistic	Cost-effective

body, are merely forms of energy. Illness and stress interrupt the free flow of energy in our bodies. Therefore, healing from a holistic perspective is about rebalancing energy.

Holism and Nursing Practice

In nursing, the root of the holistic vision and philosophy emerged from the founder of modern nursing, Florence Nightingale. Nightingale used the concept of holism and the interconnection between humans and the environment to promote healing. She not only shaped the practice of modern nursing but also made a strong differentiation between nursing and medicine. According to Nightingale (1859), medicine is a temporary process of healing; for example, surgery can simply be the removal of bullets. Neither medicine nor nursing can heal; only nature heals. Nursing, however, promotes holistic healing. All nurses have to do as health care providers is put people in the right environments with the proper nutrition, aromas, imagery, sunlight, and relaxation to promote healing (Popoola, 2003a, 2003b). To practice holistically, there must be a basic shift from the cure-driven approach of treating individual maladies to an all-inclusive focus on healing the person as a whole – body, mind, and spirit.

Nursing involvement with the practice of CAM is limited, however. It depends on licensure level and state regulations. Nurses must check with the board of nursing in their state prior to setting up independent practice that involves any form of CAM.

HOLISTIC, COMPLEMENTARY, AND ALTERNATIVE HEALING MODALITIES

Although the terms *alternative therapy* and *complementary therapy* are often interchanged, they actually refer to different concepts. Their meanings vary from culture to culture; what may be complementary in one culture may be alternative or the primary health care modality for another culture.

Complementary Versus Alternative

Nearly 40% of Americans use health care approaches outside of conventional, Western medicine (NIH, 2014a).

Complementary generally refers to using a non-mainstream approach *together with* conventional medicine.

Alternative refers to using a non-mainstream approach **in place of** conventional medicine.

True alternative medicine is not common, as most people overlap holistic therapies with conventional medicine. However, as holistic medicine becomes more mainstream, it is not unusual to find health care facilities adopting CAM therapies to help with pain management, such as guided imagery, massage, and reiki.

Integrative Medicine

According to NCCAM, integrative medicine is a growing trend among health care providers and institutions and, despite a lack of reliable, scientific data, there is emerging evidence that some of the perceived benefits are real or meaningful. In cancer treatment centers integrative health care programs offer holistic services in conjunction with chemotherapy, such as acupuncture and meditation, to manage side effects and emotional stress (National Institutes of Health [NIH], 2014a).

NCCAM uses the term "complementary health approaches" when discussing the practices and products they study, and separate the approaches into two subgroups – *natural products* and *mind and body practices.*

Natural Products

This group includes a variety of products, such as herbs (also known as botanicals), vitamins, minerals, and probiotics. They are widely marketed, readily available to consumers, and often sold as *dietary supplements.* Manufacturers of dietary supplements must comply with the 2007 FDA-issued, Good Manufacturing Practices (GMPs), which is a federal regulation for all domestic and foreign dietary supplement companies regarding their products and their distribution within the United States. Today, this regulation is known as the "Dietary Supplement Current Good Manufacturing Practices (CGMPs)" (FDA, 2014b).

Interest and use of natural products has skyrocketed in recent years with sales in the U.S. reaching an estimated 5.6 billion dollars (USD) in 2012, even though large, placebo-controlled trials have failed to show anticipated benefits. Efficacy and safety research is ongoing regarding dietary supplement reactions within the human body, along with their possible interactions with medicines and other natural products (American Botanical Council [ABC], 2013; NIH, 2014a).

Mind and Body Practices

This second NCCAM group is large and diverse, encompassing procedures or techniques that are administered or taught by a trained practitioner. Mind and body practices are designed to enhance the mind's capacity to positively affect bodily change.

- **Acupuncture** is a technique in which thin needles are inserted through the skin to stimulate specific points along an invisible energy pathway called a meridian.
- **Massage therapy** includes many different techniques in which the soft tissues of the body are manually manipulated.
- **Meditation** includes *mindfulness meditation or transcendental meditation*, and teaches focused attention.
- **Movement therapies** include a broad range of Eastern and Western movement-based approaches; examples include *Feldenkrais method, Alexander technique, Pilates, Rolfing Structural Integration, and Trager psychophysical integration.*
- **Relaxation techniques,** such as *breathing exercises, guided imagery, and progressive muscle relaxation*, assist the body's natural relaxation response.
- **Spinal manipulation** is a controlled force applied by hands or a device to a joint of the spine and is practiced by professionals such as chiropractors, osteopathic physicians,

naturopathic physicians, physical therapists, and some medical doctors.

- **Tai chi** and **qi gong** are practices from traditional Chinese medicine that combine specific movements or postures, coordinated breathing, and mental focus.
- **Yoga** includes various styles that typically combine physical postures or movement, breathing techniques, and meditation.
- **Healing touch, reiki,** and **hypnotherapy** are other examples of mind and body practices (NIH, 2014a).

CONCLUSION

*H*olism and *healing* are terms commonly used in alternative and complementary therapy. Healing is the process of becoming whole, including body, mind, and spirit. NAC therapies are used to facilitate and achieve the goals of balance, healing, and wholeness that are necessary in stress and disease management and prevention. The holistic approach to health care involves using different types of CAM or NAC therapies, behavior modification, education, and lifestyle changes. Most importantly, it requires a basic, fundamental shift from the fragmented, cure-driven approach of conventional medicine to the all-inclusive, whole body, holistic approach. Holism is an integrated and balanced lifestyle that always considers the environment, the culture, and the interconnection between humans and other forms of life and energy on Earth.

ONLINE RESOURCES

Alternative Medicine
http://www.alternativemedicine.com

Alternative Medicine Angel
http://altmedangel.com

American Music Therapy Association, Inc.
http://www.musictherapy.org

American Holistic Nurses Association
http://www.ahna.org

American Yoga Association
http://www.americanyogaassociation.org

American Association of Oriental Medicine
http://www.aaom.org

American Association of Naturopathic Physicians
http://www.naturopathic.org

Blue Poppy Press
http://www.bluepoppy.com

Center For Disease Control
http://www.cdc.gov

International Association of Interactive Imagery
http://www.iarr.org

Herbal Remedies
http://www.herbalremedies.com

Healing Touch International, Inc.
http://www.healingtouch.net

Holistic Dental Association
http://www.holisticdental.org

Holistic Networker
http://www.holisticnetworker.com

National Institute of Health
http://www.nih.gov

National Center for Complementary and Alternative Medicine
http://www.nccam.nih.gov

Nurse Healers: Professional Associates International
http://www.therapeutic-touch.org

Natural Medicines Comprehensive Database
http://www.naturaldatabase.com

World Health Organization
http://www.who.org

EXAM QUESTIONS

CHAPTER 1
Questions 1–6

Note: Choose the one option that BEST answers each question.

1. In relation to holistic healing, the acronym NAC stands for

    a. National Alternative Center.
    b. natural, alternative, and complementary.
    c. National Advocacy Center.
    d. natural alternative medicine and complementary therapy.

2. The public expressed concern over the iatrogenic effects of conventional medicines in the

    a. 1990s.
    b. 1980s.
    c. 1960s.
    d. 1940s.

3. A central theme in complementary and alternative therapy is the concept of

    a. holism.
    b. drumming.
    c. herbal therapy.
    d. aromatherapy.

4. Since illness and stress disrupt the free flow of energy in our bodies, holistic medicine

    a. is essential in traditional Western medicine.
    b. believes that healing takes place by rebalancing our energy.
    c. is a philosophy that considers some aspects of the whole person, including physical, mental, emotional, and spiritual aspects.
    d. pertains to a nursing practice directed at healing some parts of the whole person.

5. The NCCAM uses the term "complementary health approaches" to describe the two subgroups they study. One subgroup is

    a. mind and body practices.
    b. biofeedback.
    c. meditation.
    d. dance.

6. Mind and body medicine uses a variety of techniques designed to enhance the mind's capacity, such as

    a. shark cartilage and chelation therapies.
    b. occupational and physical therapy.
    c. meditation, yoga, and guided imagery.
    d. dietary supplements.

CHAPTER 2

COMMON TYPES OF COMPLEMENTARY AND ALTERNATIVE THERAPIES

CHAPTER OBJECTIVE

Upon completion of this chapter, the learner will be able to recognize the various types of commonly used holistic, natural, alternative, and complementary healing therapies.

LEARNING OBJECTIVES

After studying this chapter, the learner will be able to:

1. Describe the types of complementary therapies commonly used in the United States.
2. Indicate the differences between massage therapy and Therapeutic Touch or reflexology.
3. Differentiate the various commonly used complementary therapies.

INTRODUCTION

The holistic natural, alternative, and complementary (NAC) therapies that are commonly used today in the United States are defined and discussed briefly below. Most of these therapies are discussed in more detail in later chapters. It should be noted, however, that the identification and use of NAC therapies in the United States is still evolving.

Types of complementary and alternative therapy that will be discussed in this chapter are

- herbal therapy
- aromatherapy
- massage therapy
- reflexology
- music therapy
- Therapeutic Touch
- yoga
- meditation
- aquatic therapy
- African folk healing practices
- prayer and spiritual healing practices
- homeopathy
- acupuncture
- Chinese medicine
- exercise therapy
- humor and laughter therapy
- relaxation exercises
- guided imagery
- nutrition therapy.

HERBAL THERAPY

Herbal therapy is the use of an herb or any part of a plant for culinary or medicinal purposes. Herbal therapies are also sometimes referred to as "botanicals," "nutraceuticals," or "phytomedicines." Dietary supplements are considered a part of herbal therapy.

Until the 1950s, the United States federal government regulated herbs as drugs. For example, in 1938, the U.S. Food and Drug Administration passed the Food, Drug, and Cosmetic Act, which required all drugs, including herbs, to be proven safe before they could be sold. In 1962, the Food, Drug, and Cosmetic Act was amended by the Kefauver-Harris Drug Amendments, which required manufacturers to also prove to the FDA the effectiveness of drugs and herbs before they could be marketed (Lilley & Aucker, 2003).

Parts of herbs used in herbal therapies include leaves, flowers, fruits, seeds, stems, wood, bark, roots, and rhizomes. Herbal remedies are dispensed as brews and powders and can be used in cooking or making drinks. Herbalists known as *shamans,* or traditional healers, also make ointments and poultices out of herbs.

Herbal therapy has been the core of most systems of medicine from the beginning of civilization, and herbs are quickly becoming one of the most commonly used NAC therapies. Some commonly used herbs with therapeutic value are echinacea (immune stimulant and anti-infection agent); garlic (antihypertensive and antibiotic); ginger (antinauseant and antispasmodic); ginseng root (increased stamina and decreased fatigue); kava kava (calming effect); and St. John's wort (anxiolytic and antidepressant).

AROMATHERAPY

Aromatherapy involves the use of essential oils (extracts or essences) from flowers, herbs, and trees to promote health and well-being. In the past decade, most people have turned to NAC therapies, such as aromatherapy, to treat stress and relieve disease symptoms. Essential oils can be used in a variety of therapeutic ways. In addition, many essential oils are potent antibiotic agents. Aromatherapy can also be used to promote sleep, alleviate anxiety or pain, and improve mood. Although the psychological benefits of aromatherapy have been shown, the physiological benefits of essential oils, specifically their antibacterial effects, are still debatable. Two classical essential oils are lavender and peppermint. Lavender is used to reduce stress and depression and promote relaxation; peppermint is used to treat headaches, digestive disorders, and muscle aches.

MASSAGE THERAPY

Massage therapy is the manipulation of muscle and connective tissue to enhance function and promote relaxation and well-being. It is an alternative and complementary healing modality with an ancient history. Massage therapy can be as simple as a back rub performed by a trained nurse or as complex as sustained light and deep tissue massage performed by a massage therapist. Different types of massage therapy and techniques exist. Massage therapy can include pressing, rubbing, pulling, staccato touch, light touch, gliding strokes, matching, back walking, kneading, tapping, shaking, and cupping. These various techniques are practiced differently from culture to culture and may be given different names.

REFLEXOLOGY

Reflexology involves the use of different massage and pressure techniques to relax and loosen muscles in the feet and hands. Reflexology is based on the concept that energy zones connect certain areas of the body to the feet and hands. In this way, the feet and hands are viewed as maps or mirrors of the body. Putting pressure on and massaging specific points on the feet or hands is believed to affect the corresponding area of the body. Each foot contains more than 7,000 nerve endings. Technically, foot massage with a clear intention to manipulate these nerve endings is a form of reflexology. To an extent, reflexology can be performed on oneself.

MUSIC THERAPY

Music therapy is the use of music to promote healing and enrich our lives. Music makes us smile, laugh, dance, and cry. It stirs up deep reservoirs of feeling, transcends time, and provides a sense of well-being. There is evidence that music therapy can help to reduce pain, relieve stress and anxiety, encourage emotional expression and promote social interaction (American Cancer Society [ACS], 2014a).

The evolution of music as a therapy has been based on the healing practices of many cultures. In the 1940s, music therapy was first used with patients in psychiatric hospitals. The American Music Therapy Association was founded in 1998 for the purpose of developing music therapy for use in rehabilitation, special education, and community health care settings. Music therapy offers an array of benefits, with virtually no risks to clients. Music is used to enhance physical, psychological, cognitive, and social functioning for patients of all ages and cultures.

THERAPEUTIC TOUCH

Therapeutic Touch, a contemporary interpretation of several ancient healing practices, is a scientifically based practice founded on the premise that the body, mind, emotions, and spirit form a complex, dynamic energy field. The practice was developed by Dolores Krieger, a professor of nursing at New York University, and Dora Van Gelder Kunz, a natural healer. Therapeutic Touch is based on a belief in universal energy flow and human energy fields; these energy fields flow in balanced patterns in health but are depleted or unbalanced in illness or injury. In the practice of Therapeutic Touch, a practitioner uses his or her hands to intentionally direct energy exchange in such a way as to facilitate the healing process.

YOGA

Yoga is a unique holistic practice and way of life that incorporates meditation, poses (asanas), and breathing. It is a psychophysiological discipline with roots that date back 5,000 years. Founded by Patanjali, the practice includes standing, sitting, balancing, and breathing poses, as well as twists and inversion movements, each designed to offer particular health and spiritual benefits. By controlling breathing and holding the body in steady poses, yoga creates body, mind, and spirit harmony and promotes relaxation.

MEDITATION

Meditation is the art of focusing attention so completely on one thing that everything else around it loses substance. Meditation has a religious and philosophical background. Although it can be used alone, it is frequently used with relaxation exercises, yoga, and other types of alternative therapies. With meditation, we can learn to control our bodies; it is like the experience we have in a movie theater when we stay focused. It is a very effective method of relaxation. Unlike hypnosis, which is a passive experience, meditation is an active process directed toward balancing the mind, body, and spirit.

AQUATIC THERAPY

Aquatic therapy, also called *hydrotherapy,* entails a purposeful progression of motor skills focusing on psychosocial, cognitive, leisure, and motor performance using the properties of water to enhance the benefits of the experience. Aquatic therapy can be done independently, in a group setting, or with a therapist to increase an individual's physical, social, cognitive, spiritual, and social domain.

Evidence of aquatic therapy dates back to the fifth century B.C. In the river valleys of

Mesopotamia, Egypt, India, and China, bath pools and spas were used for social, spiritual, and healing purposes. Healing water rituals also appear in ancient Greek, Hebrew, Roman, Christian, and Islamic cultures, in which water was used to cleanse the physical body of diseases and the spiritual body of sin. For example, the island Bimini in the Bahamas, located 50 miles from Miami, is famous for its legendary "Fountain of Youth," with its healing waters.

AFRICAN FOLK HEALING PRACTICES

In almost every traditional culture, symbolic rituals, such as dance are a part of the process of healing. Although the meanings of such rituals may vary from culture to culture, the symbolic meaning remains a reminder that life can be fragile. One such healing practice common in Africa and the Caribbean is the process of breaking and sharing cola nut, coconut, or any other nut as a symbolic gesture. Parts of such nuts are frequently offered to Mother Earth, representing that, in times of happiness, wholeness, and peace, some evil force may want to break us or take our wholeness away by disconnecting us from our balance (earth). Giving back part of the nut to the earth shows willingness to give something back during difficult and stressful times in our lives to regain that balance. The cola nut is used symbolically in Nigeria for most healing and cultural events and has become a metaphor for holism, peace, and healing. Prayer, meditation, herbs, imagery, dancing, and drumming are also African folk healing practices.

PRAYER AND SPIRITUAL HEALING PRACTICES

Although traditional and spiritual healers are common in every culture, their practices may vary slightly from culture to culture. Spiritual healers may also go by such names as herbalist, voodoo, native doctor, wise man, shaman, and priest. However, the concept of "spiritual healer" discussed here refers to a person who heals by prayers and by faith with clear intentions for healing. The use of prayer and spiritual healing is not new to any society; however, its use in modern nursing and medical practice is new. Spiritual healing usually involves praying for or with someone, "laying on of the hands" for spiritual blessings, distance prayer and healing, or symbolic rituals such as the cross or rosary. Personal prayers can instill hope and reduce the anxieties associated with illness and other stressors.

HOMEOPATHY

Homeopathy is strongly rooted in the belief that the body has the capacity to heal itself. Unlike conventional medicine, which focuses on suppressing bodily responses and replacing substances that the body has failed to produce or using small doses of disease-producing agents to sensitize or desensitize the immune system, homeopathic medicine initiates the body's return to a state of balance (homeostasis). Homeopathic remedies and medicines are usually manufactured from natural substances, such as plants, metals, minerals, venoms, animals, and even bacteria.

ACUPUNCTURE

Acupuncture is the practice of inserting needles into specific exterior body locations to relieve pain, induce surgical anesthesia, and achieve other therapeutic goals. The practice of acupuncture originated in China. The needles used in this practice can be sharp, round, blunt, three-edged, swordlike, or sharp-round filiform and are used to manipulate various acupuncture points or meridians in the body.

CHINESE MEDICINE

According to Chinese culture, everyone is born with a self-healing ability and the body has the ability to regenerate its immune system. The human body is an organic whole with an inseparable connection to the natural world and the universe as a whole. In addition, the Chinese believe that destructive energy patterns, such as cancer, can be interrupted and broken by the balance of yin and yang, a key philosophy of Chinese medicine. The best cure in Chinese practice is prevention. The Chinese believe that the body has five main centers: heart/mind, lungs, liver, spleen, and kidneys. They believe there are six external disease-causing factors: wind, cold, heat, moisture, dryness, and fire. They also believe there are seven emotions: happiness, anger, worry, pensiveness, grief, fear, and surprise. Balancing these emotions is critical in the Chinese healing practice.

EXERCISE THERAPY

Exercise therapy is the use of a muscle or part of the body in a repetitive way for the beneficial purpose of improving, developing, or maintaining body strength, maintaining fitness, conditioning the body, improving health, correcting deformities, restoring body systems or organs to a state of wellness, and encouraging relaxation. Exercise therapy can be active or passive, isometric or isotonic, aerobic or anaerobic, and progressive or steady range of motion. It can also be combined with aquatic therapy.

Exercise therapy is a very common NAC therapy that has been proven to

- lower cholesterol
- lower blood pressure
- improve sleep
- boost confidence
- improve body circulation

- protect the body against injury and disease
- reduce stress and tension
- make bones stronger
- improve posture
- increase oxygen to the bones and muscles.

For the purpose of this book, the type of exercise therapy that will be focused on is relaxation exercise. Relaxation is a change and relief from effort, work, and tension.

RELAXATION EXERCISES

Tension can lead to emotional, physical, psychological, spiritual, and economic imbalances that can lead to disease. Relaxation exercise is a commonly used intervention for anxious patients. Relaxation exercise has many forms; most relaxation exercise includes breathing exercises. Relaxation activities can bring back balance and peace, which can facilitate healing. Relaxation of the body, mind, and spirit can create a state of wholeness and reduce stress, and it is the most cost-effective way to promote self-healing.

HUMOR AND LAUGHTER THERAPY

As the old saying goes, laughter is good medicine. Just as exercise can strengthen the body and invigorate the spirit, scientists believe that laughter and humor can be physically and emotionally therapeutic. Laughter has potential healing and preventative effects on our health. It can

- relax the muscles
- reduce pain
- relieve stress
- optimize immune system function
- lower blood pressure
- improve circulation
- diffuse anger.

Humor and laughter have long been used to cope with illness and stress. In fact, the practice dates back to biblical days. For example, Proverbs 17:22 notes that a cheerful heart does good like a medicine but a broken spirit makes one sick. Humor and laugher therapy are separate practices but are often used in conjunction.

GUIDED IMAGERY

Guided imagery is a therapeutic technique for promoting relaxation and relieving pain in which the patient is encouraged to concentrate on or visualize an image. Imagery carries extraordinary power. Every time someone asks, "Do you remember the time when...?" it acts as a vehicle to bring a certain image to bear, flooding us with some association that enables or pushes us to remember the experience. Directing the minds to the inner world of memories, fantasies, dreams, and visions can help us transcend the worries of life and provide us with a tool for self-healing. Guided imagery is a tool that can be used to connect the body, mind and spirit to help us achieve holism.

NUTRITION THERAPY

Like herbal therapy, nutrition therapy is a commonly used NAC therapeutic modality. Nutrition therapy and diet modification are about mind over matter (body). They involve a holistic balance of life and diet that focuses on taking care of oneself. No medications, special diets, or health practitioners can achieve that goal for a person. Some diets have side effects, lack balanced nutrition, encourage lack of self-control on the part of the patient, and focus on curing (the medical model), which is temporary. It is common knowledge that most people who lose weight using a rigid diet plan are likely to gain it back, and possibly more, once they stop using the diet plan.

For nutrition therapy to be effective and long lasting, people must be willing to control and manage what they eat as well as change their philosophy of life. There is no magic "cure" when it comes to obesity. Nutrition therapy is about learning to live holistically and taking care of oneself from a holistic self-care approach. The abundance of information available today about nutrition and dieting could be overwhelming even to a rocket scientist. The bottom line is that to lose 1 lb, a person must decrease his or her food intake by 3,500 calories or increase exercise or energy loss by the same amount. This could take days, weeks, or months. However, it is much easier to put on weight. Some supersized fast-food meals alone have approximately 3,500 calories! A holistic diet focuses on balancing homeostasis and understanding that food cravings and overeating have an emotional component and a physiological side effect – overweight or obesity.

CONCLUSION

Regardless of the stressors in our daily life and the illnesses we are battling, NAC therapies, such as herbal therapy, aromatherapy, massage therapy, reflexology, music therapy, Therapeutic Touch, yoga, meditation, aquatic therapy, African folk healing practices, prayer and spiritual healing, homeopathy, acupuncture, Chinese medicine, exercise and relaxation therapy, humor and laughter therapy, guided imagery, and nutrition therapy can always be used to help us achieve and maintain a sense of balance and homeostasis. Health care providers, especially nurses, can be influential in teaching patients the practice of holistic and self-care approaches to healing. Many of the different types of complementary and alternative therapies presented in this chapter can be used today to achieve healing and prevent chronic illnesses.

ONLINE RESOURCES

Alternative Medicine Angel
   http://www.altmedangel.com

Aquatic Resources Network
   http://www.aquaticnet.com/index.htm

American Music Therapy Association, Inc.
   http://www.musictherapy.org

A World of Yoga
   http://www.yogaworld.org

International Association of Interactive Imagery
   http://www.iarr.org

Holistic online
   http://www.holistic-online.com

Holistic Networker
   http://www.holisticnetworker.com

Holistic Healing
   http://www.healing.about.com

The Transcendent Meditation Program
   http://www.tm.org

The Watsu Institute
   http://www.watsu.com

Yoga Directory
   http://www.yogadirectory.com

EXAM QUESTIONS

CHAPTER 2
Questions 7–13

Note: Choose the one option that BEST answers each question.

7. The NAC therapy that involves the use of essential oils is

   a. massage.

   b. yoga.

   c. aromatherapy.

   d. herbal therapy.

8. The NAC therapy that involves massage and pressure techniques to relax and loosen muscles in the feet and hands is called

   a. massage.

   b. reflexology.

   c. meditation.

   d. hypnosis.

9. The NAC therapy or practice developed by Dolores Krieger and Dora Van Gelder Kunz is called

   a. aquatic therapy.

   b. African folk healing practice.

   c. Therapeutic Touch.

   d. homeopathy.

10. Needles are inserted into specific exterior body locations to relieve pain, induce surgical anesthesia, and achieve other therapeutic goals in the NAC therapy known as

    a. massage.

    b. reflexology.

    c. meditation.

    d. acupuncture.

11. The concept of yin and yang originated from

    a. African healing practices.

    b. Japanese medicine.

    c. Native American healing practices.

    d. Chinese medicine.

12. The most cost-effective NAC healing practice is

    a. herbal therapy.

    b. massage.

    c. relaxation.

    d. music therapy.

13. To lose 1 lb, a person must decrease food intake by

    a. 2,500 calories.

    b. 3,500 calories.

    c. 4,500 calories.

    d. 5,500 calories.

CHAPTER 3

AROMATHERAPY

CHAPTER OBJECTIVE

Upon completion of this chapter, the learner will be able to discuss the history, properties, and actions of aromatherapy and its uses as a holistic alternative and complementary therapy.

LEARNING OBJECTIVES

After studying this chapter, the learner will be able to:

1. Describe the history of aromatherapy use.
2. Identify common methods of extracting different types of essential oils.
3. Differentiate between the various methods of preparing and administering aromatherapy.
4. List the benefits of aromatherapy as a holistic alternative and complementary therapy.
5. Identify at least ten of the most common essential oils and their aromas.
6. Discuss the different uses of aromatherapy to achieve healing.
7. Discuss the nursing responsibilities and implications associated with aromatherapy use.

INTRODUCTION

In the past decade, many people have turned to complementary and alternative medicine (CAM) to prevent and manage stress and diseases. Aromatherapy, an example of one of these CAM therapies, is the use of essential oils to achieve a desired effect that is often therapeutic.

Since our earliest history, humans have mined the sensory pleasures and medicinal powers of plants, flowers, herbs, roots, and trees. These botanicals are the core of the ancient practice of aromatherapy. Essential oils (extracts or essences) and aromatherapy are used not only to enhance healing but also to promote health and well-being and for cosmetic purposes. For example, aromatherapy can be used to promote sleep, alleviate anxiety or pain, and improve mood. Some oils have also been used as potent antibiotic agents. Although the psychological benefits of aromatherapy have been shown, the physiological benefits of essential oils, specifically their antibacterial effects, are still debatable.

This chapter discusses the use of aromatherapy as a holistic therapeutic modality and natural, alternative, and complementary (NAC) therapy. Common essential oils and their uses are described. In addition, the chapter details the history of aromatherapy use.

DESCRIPTION OF AROMATHERAPY

The National Association for Holistic Aromatherapy (NAHA) defines *aromatherapy* as "the art and science of utilizing naturally extracted aromatic essences from plants to balance, harmonize, and promote the health of body, mind, and spirit" (NAHA, 2014a). This holistic practice seeks to enhance the physiological, psychological, and spiritual realms of the human response to aromatic extracts and their innate healing abilities (NAHA, 2014a).

Aromatherapy uses fragrant essences found in all parts of the plant: blossoms, berries, fruits, seeds, pods, stems, leaves, needles, bark, rind, resin, wood, and roots. When the plant essences are naturally distilled or mechanically pressed, without chemical processes, they become true essential oils. These oils are very concentrated, volatile, and evaporate quickly when exposed to air. Each type of essential oil is chemically different, even oils from plants within the same species or those that are grown or harvested in different ways or locations (NIH, 2012).

As a holistic therapy, aromatherapy has both preventative and active treatment properties that can be beneficial during periods of wellness as well as during acute and chronic stages of illness or disease. Cerrato (1998) and Nelson (1997) note that the holistic value of aromatherapy cannot be underestimated.

Essential oils are the foundation of aromatherapy. The use of essential oils is a natural, noninvasive treatment modality that affects the whole person, not just the symptom or disease. This practice is used to enhance the body's natural ability to balance, regulate, heal, and maintain itself through the use of specific essential oils. The aroma of light oils from flowers, plants, and seeds are used to pamper tired muscles and uplift moods, and herbal infusions are often used to invigorate, stimulate, and rejuvenate the spirit and to relieve deep worries and stress. Aromatherapy is also used to manage many chronic health problems A leading theory about how aromatherapy works is that when we breathe in the scents of essential oils, olfactory receptors in the nose transmit chemical messages to the brain's limbic system, which affects moods and emotions. Imaging studies in humans have shown how smells affect the limbic system

and its emotional pathways (NIH, 2012). Aromatherapy is essentially an interaction between the therapist, the client, and essential oils in which healing energy is brought forth to help the client regain his or her sense of well-being and vitality (Kusmirek, 1998).

HISTORY OF AROMATHERAPY

Aromatherapy is as old as humanity itself. Aromatherapy is the relationship of the natural world and the five human senses. For thousands of years, plants and flowers have been used to heal humans. In fact, in prehistoric times, humans were able to recognize the various scents nature provided from animals, plants, flowers, trees, grains, roots, and resins and they relied on their sense of smell to survive. Later, they discovered the medicinal values of spices and herbs. Plants and essences played a very important role in the healing, spiritual, secular, and cosmetic practices of the ancient Egyptians, Chinese, Greeks, Romans, and Indians (aworldofaromatherapy.com, n.d.). The early aromatherapists in all cultures were priests, gods, and goddesses. Aromatherapy and some of the early popular aromas, such as frankincense and myrrh, are still used today in many of these cultures.

The Origins of Aromatherapy

The Egyptians were the first true aromatherapists, having used the practice as far back as 6000 B.C. for religious and medicinal purposes as well as in embalming, perfumes, incenses, fragrances, and cosmetics (Bright, 2002; Thomas, 2002). However, the Israelites, Greeks, Romans, Arabs, Indians, Chinese, and Europeans also used aromatherapy. The use of aromatherapy has even spread to the American public over the last two centuries.

In the Chinese culture, aromatherapy dates back to 2700 B.C., when more than 300 plants were documented in an herbal book by the Chinese Emperor Shen Nung. However, it was the Greek alchemists who invented and used distillation of plant materials with water, and eventually alcohol, to extract essential oils. Distillation of essential oils has provided one of the most sophisticated paths to pleasure known to mankind in all cultures. Improving on the work of the Greeks, the Romans expanded the use of aromas and created what was known as the "Bath Capital of the World." The Romans not only added essential oils to their baths but also used them for massage therapy after their baths. They later exported their bath and massage oils to other countries.

The actual practice of aromatherapy is credited to Rene Maurice Gattefosse. a French chemist who was the first person to transform the practice from an anecdotal science to a well-recognized NAC therapy. In 1930, Gattefosse coined the term *aromatherapy*. He discovered the benefits of lavender oil when it healed his burned hand without leaving any scars (aworldofaromatherapy.com, n.d.).

Aromatherapy and Nursing

In nursing, the use of aromatherapy can be traced back as early as 1859 when Florence Nightingale made use of the practice. Like Hippocrates, the father of modern medicine, Nightingale often talked about the use of aromatherapy in her practice. She burned rosemary and lavender for fumigation of the streets and hospitals. In her book *Notes on Nursing*, Nightingale (1859) advocated for the use of different types of essential oils to create a healing environment and to promote healing in individuals, communities, hospital environments, and homes. According to Stevensen (1998) and Thomas (2002), this trend continued into the 1980s, with increasing research on the clinical effectiveness of aromatherapy.

AROMATHERAPY PRACTICE

Aromatherapy is based on the idea that boosting the body's defense mechanisms and immune system via touch and smell can promote and maintain health. This therapeutic modality helps restore harmony and energy balance between the body, mind, spirit, and outside world – a harmony that is continually disrupted by pollution, stress, busy schedules, pathogens, diseases, and the other rigors of modern life. Essential oils stimulate the powerful sense of smell and operate on the basic premise that one of the functions of the sense of smell is to connect our body to our mind (brain) via the olfactory nerves. The olfactory, or smell, center in the limbic system is also located with the emotion center in the brain. These smell and emotion centers bypass the cognitive center. Therefore, the brain selectively responds to various emotions and senses with and without our awareness. This powerful sense of smell allows essential oils to stimulate and produce various emotions. This explains how aromatherapy works and why pleasant-smelling botanical oils, such as lavender, rose, lemon, and peppermint, are widely used for their relaxing and calming effects.

Most essential oils have a variety of properties. Some act as antiseptic, antiviral, anti-inflammatory, analgesic, antidepressant, decongestant, or expectorant agents, whereas others have stimulating, soothing, refreshing, calming, balancing, harmonizing, uplifting, sedating, rejuvenating, toning, warming, cooling, or relaxing effects. Certain oils can also be used to improve digestion, promote concentration, boost the immune system, assist diuresis, dispel fears, and enhance sensuality (Thomas, 2002). Essential oils are generally dynamic, active, and highly sensitive substances that act quickly when applied to the body, diffusing through the skin and penetrating blood vessel walls and body tissues. Therefore, essential oils should be used and handled with caution.

Aromatherapy Oils

Essential oils are complex organic chemicals that are soluble in vegetable oil and alcohol. People can smell the aroma of essential oils because these oils are natural chemical substances that evaporate quickly when exposed to air. These oils are also highly volatile substances that contain hydrogen, carbon, and oxygen. Chemically, the primary functional groups of essential oils used in aromatherapy are monoterpenes, esters, aldehydes, ketones, alcohols, phenols, and oxides (BioSpiritual Energy Healing, n.d.).

Each essential oil has its own special scent and healing properties. Hundreds of essential oils are available on the market today. According to the NAHA (2014c), the most commonly used essential oils are:

Roman chamomile (*Chamaemelum nobile*): antispasmodic, menstrual cramps, sedative, relieves anxiety/stress, insomnia, anti-inflammatory

Clary sage (*Salvia sclarea*): antispasmodic, relieves menstrual cramps, aphrodisiac, relaxing, relieves anxiety/stress, labor pain management

Eucalyptus globulus: expectorant, decongestant, beneficial for flu/cold season, clearing to the mind, energizing, bronchitis (**avoid with children under 2**)

Eucalyptus radiata: expectorant, useful for colds and flu, antiviral

Fennel (*Foeniculum vulgare var. dulce*): digestive, menstrual irregularities, antimicrobial

Frankincense (*Boswellia frereana*): strengthens the immune system (CO_2 extract), soothes inflamed skin conditions, cell regenerative

Geranium (*Pelargonium x asperum syn. graveolens*): PMS, indicated for hormonal imbalance, antimicrobial, nerve pain

Ginger (*Zingiber officinale*): digestive, useful to eliminate gas, constipation, relieves nausea, warming emotionally and physically, anti-inflammatory, relieves pain, immune modulator

Helichrysum (*Helichrysum italicum*): cell regenerative, wound healing, anti-inflammatory, indicated for bruises and swelling

Lavender (*Lavandula angustifolia*): calming, reduces anxiety, wound healing, burns, cell regenerative, insect bites. reduces itchiness, general skin care, antispasmodic

Lemon (*Citrus limon*): antiviral, great for cleaning home, cleansing to environments (room spray), uplifting, detoxing

Lemongrass (*Cymbopogon citratus*): cleansing, antiviral, insect repellant, use for cleaning, antimicrobial

Mandarin (*Citrus reticulata*): calming, (can combine with lavender), slightly more warming citrus aroma

Neroli (*Citrus aurantium var. amara*): relieves and reduces anxiety, antispasmodic, PMS, antidepressant, nourishing, postpartum depression, pregnancy/delivery

Patchouli (*Pogostemom cablin*): antidepressant, anti-inflammatory, soothes the nervous system

Peppermint (*Mentha x piperita*): relieves nausea, analgesic for muscular aches and pains, relieves/reduces migraines, energizing, antispasmodic, **do not use on children under 30 months of age**

(NAHA, 2014c)

More information is presented in Table 3-1.

Name	Aroma	Use
Basil (*Ocimum basilicum*)	Sweet and spicy	Antispasmodic used for respiratory tract infections, asthma, bronchitis and digestive disorders; uplifting, refreshing oil that also aids concentration
Clary sage (*Salvia sclarea*)	Herbaceous and floral	Warming, relaxing, uplifting, calming, soothing, anticonvulsant, antidepressant, bactericidal, antiseptic properties that are useful for menstrual problems, depression, asthma, whooping cough, colic, cramps, and amenorrhea
Eucalyptus (*Eucalyptus globulus* or *Eucalyptus radiate*)	Strong	Head-clearing and invigorating; also antiseptic and decongestant; helpful in treating respiratory problems, such as coughs, colds, and asthma; helps to boost the immune system; and relieves muscle tension
Geranium (*Pelargonium graveolens*)	Fruity	Used to balance hormones in women and balance skin tone, can be both relaxing and uplifting; also used as an antidepressant
Grapefruit (*Citrus paradise*)	Sweet, citrusy, fruity, sharp, and refreshing	Relaxing, calming, and uplifting
Jasmine (*Jasminium grandiflorum* or *officinale*)	Exotic, rich, sweet, and floral	Relaxing, soothing stimulant with mild analgesic, antidepressant, antiseptic, antispasmodic, aphrodisiac, sedative, and expectorant properties
Lavender (*Lavandula angustifolia*)	Herbaceous and floral	Sedative used for stress reduction, calming, and depression; also used for skin care and in treatment of burns and wounds; refreshing, relaxing, calming, soothing oil with therapeutic qualities
Lemon (*Citrus limon*)	Fresh, sharp, citrusy, and stimulating	Very uplifting, yet relaxing and sedating; commonly used for anxiety and is helpful in treating wounds, infections, and inflammation; also used for house cleaning and deodorizing
Lemon balm (*Melissa officinalis*)	Fresh and sharp	Used for excitability, dementia, restlessness, anxiety, stress, and insomnia; refreshing, stimulating, uplifting, and motivating
Orange (*Citrus sinensis*)	Fresh, sharp, citrusy, and stimulating	Refreshing, relaxing, and very stimulating
Peppermint (*Mentha piperita*)	Minty and strong	Used to treat headaches, muscle aches, and digestive disorders such as slow digestion; excellent for indigestion and flatulence
Roman chamomile (*Anthemidis*)	Refreshing	Very relaxing oil that can help with sleeplessness, anxiety, muscle aches, and tension; also used to treat wounds and infection
Rosemary (*Rosmarinus officinalis*)	Refreshing	Stimulating, invigorating, clarifying, and uplifting; stimulates cognitive status and the immune and digestive systems; good for muscle aches and tension
Tea tree (*Melaleuca alternifolia*)	Strong, medicinal, eucalyptus-like, and refreshing	Well known for its antibacterial action; used for wound healing and antiseptic purposes and to strengthen or boost the immune system; also considered a natural antifungal, good for treating all sorts of fungal infections including vaginal yeast infections, jock itch, athletes' foot, and ringworm
Thyme (*Thymus vulgaris*)	Stimulating, refreshing, and sharp	Antiseptic and strong bactericidal; refreshing, strengthens the immune system; used for cough or as a lip balm
Ylang-ylang (*Cananga odorata*)	Fresh	Used to relax and reduce muscle tension; also a good antidepressant

(Holistic-online.com, n.d.-b)

Although the majority are used for general therapeutic and cosmetic purposes, in many cultures some are valued for their medicinal and antibiotic properties. Types of aromatherapy products that can be purchased are ointments, lotions, creams, soaps, presses, vaporizers, incense, and candles.

Penetration: Essential oils enter the body via the skin and nose. When the tiny molecules are massaged into the skin, they penetrate the bloodstream and act on the organs within the body, creating an extraordinary physiological effect.

Inhalation: Inhaling natural substances is an exquisite, complex, profound, seductive, mysterious, and primitive experience. Whether essential oils are burned and infused into the atmosphere, applied to certain body parts, or simply inhaled, a significant concentration of odor molecules reaches the olefactory receptors. It has also been anecdotally reported that inhaled essential oils alter the chemistry of the body and cause mind-altering effects when they penetrate the bloodstream and reach the limbic center of the brain.

Use of Touch: When essential oils are gently massaged into the skin, the nervous system is stimulated, the internal organs are treated, the senses are awakened, the emotions are soothed, and the spirit soars. This is a very comforting and caring intervention produced not only by the touch but also by the aroma of the essential oil.

Methods of Extracting Essential Oils

True essential oils are extracted from the barks, roots, berries, flowers, stalks, leaves, and resins of trees and plants. For an essential oil to be a true essential oil, it must be isolated by physical means. Below are some of the processes by which these essential oils can be extracted. These processes are also summarized in Table 3-2.

TABLE 3-2: METHODS OF EXTRACTING ESSENTIAL OILS

Steam distillation: Most common form of extracting essential oils

Maceration: Labor intensive and costly method of extracting essential oils

Enfleurage: Used when the flower oils are too delicate or fugitive to undergo distillation

Expression: Used exclusively to extract essential oils from citrus fruits; also known as *cold pressing*

Solvent extraction: May or may not affect the aroma or therapeutic benefits

Synthetics: The process of making essential oils without using the real ingredients in an organic process

---

Steam Distillation

Steam distillation is the most common method of extracting essential oils that are contained in the glands, veins, sacs, and glandular hairs of aromatic plants. Steam extraction occurs when the cell walls of these plants are ruptured by heat. The molecules are carried in the steam through a pipe. As they cool and condense, the essential oil separates from the water.

Maceration

Maceration is a labor-intensive and costly method of extracting essential oils. Sometimes compared to the digestion of food, the process involves steeping the plant in a liquid in order to extract soluble constituents or to soften, separate, or break the molecules. It may or may not involve heat. This process is not commonly used. Examples of oils extracted by maceration are onion, garlic, wintergreen, and bitter almond.

Enfleurage

Enfleurage involves impregnating or soaking plants in warm, nonodorous oils until their precious essential oils are expressed into the carrier oil. This process is used when the flower oils are too delicate or short-lived to undergo distillation.

Expression

Expression is a method used exclusively to extract essential oils from citrus fruits. When the peel of such a fruit is mechanically pressed, droplets of oil and juice are squeezed out and separated. This method is also known as *cold pressing.*

Solvent Extraction

In solvent extraction, aromatic compounds are extracted using hydrocarbon solvents. Solvent-extracted scents, or fragrances, always have a slight petroleum smell, which may or may not affect their aromas or therapeutic benefits.

Synthetics

Synthetic production uses organic chemistry to create essential oils in the laboratory that have synthetic smells. Simply stated, it is the process of making essential oils without using the real ingredients. Note, however, that when it comes to healing, naturally made essential oils are considered more useful than synthetic products because synthetics may lack some of the harmonic and healing properties of the natural products.

Benefits of Aromatherapy

The NAHA classifies aromatherapy as a holistic therapy that can be used at several levels for physiological, psychological, spiritual, and preventive healing and for acute and chronic problems. It can also be used to promote health and well-being. The use of aromatherapy for the management of acute or chronic pain is thought to work by enhancing the parasympathetic response through the effects of touch and relaxation (George & Minski, 1996; Kacperek, 1997; Stevensen, 1998). Relaxation is a common use for essential oils. Table 3-3 presents some essential oils that can be used for relaxation. Specifically, essential oils can be used to

TABLE 3-3: ESSENTIAL OILS USEFUL FOR RELAXATION	
• Basil	• Lemongrass
• Cedarwood	• Melissa
• Clary sage	• Myrrh
• Clove	• Orange
• Cypress	• Peppermint
• Eucalyptus	• Roman chamomile
• Frankincense	• Rosemary
• Ginger	• Rosewood
• Grapefruit	• Sandalwood
• Jasmine	• Tea tree
• Lavender	• Thyme
• Lemon	• Ylang-ylang

calm or uplift the spirit. They can also be used for wound healing and treatment of infections (Stevensen, 1998). Essential oils are sometimes used with a variety of other types of NAC therapies, most commonly with massage therapy but also with aquatic therapy in aromatherapy baths.

As a holistic modality or therapy, aromatherapy has both preventative and healing qualities. These qualities have resulted in increased recognition over the years, making aromatherapy one of the fastest growing NAC therapies. For example, the American Cancer Society has approved the use of complementary therapies, including aromatherapy, when used with standard medical treatment to help relieve cancer symptoms and side effects of chemotherapy, ease pain and nausea, and improve quality of life in cancer patients (Fellowes, Barnes, & Wilkinson, 2004). As a natural, noninvasive treatment, aromatherapy and essential oils can be used for medicinal, spiritual, and cosmetic purposes. Specifically, essential oils can be used to treat physiological problems, including nausea, arthritis, chronic pain, and reproductive health problems, such as premenstrual syndrome, vaginitis, and menopause (Buckle, 1999; Rose, 2001); for psychological problems, such as depression, anxiety, and dementia (Ballard, O'Brien, Reichelt, & Perry, 2002), and for spiritual reasons (Thomas, 2002; Buckle, 1999). Aromatherapy can also be used to enrich the immune system; treat upper respiratory tract symptoms; improve memory; alleviate stress and fears; promote sedation; treat common skin conditions, such as acne and sun burns; and treat infections, such as sinusitis. Table 3-4 lists just some of the numerous indications for essential oil use. *Note:* For a more comprehensive list of indications, actions, companion oils and cautions, please go to http://www.natural-holistic-health.com/single-essential-oil-profiles

Methods of Administering Essential Oils

Essential oils are easy to use. For example, they can be used by simply adding them to a bath basin or a foot soak. However, certain methods of administration are recommended for therapeutic benefits (Bright, 2002).

Although almost all essential oils can be absorbed into the body via the skin (direct topical administration), only certain essential oils (for example, lavender and tea tree oils) should be placed directly on the skin. Inhalation is generally considered the safest, most understood method of administering and using essential oils. In addition, inhalation via the olfactory or limbic system is considered the fastest route of administration. Aromatherapy can also be administered orally, rectally, vaginally, topically via massage, or by diffusion in the air.

Essential oils may be blended into a base of carrier oil or diluted for various therapeutic and clinical purposes. Some examples of carrier oils are sweet almond, grape seed, calendula, hazelnut, sesame seed, and avocado. It should be noted that people without training or

---

TABLE 3-4: INDICATIONS FOR AROMATHERAPY

Emotional
- Depression or hopelessness
- Frustration
- Anxiety or nervous tension
- Insomnia
- Lack of concentration
- Irritability
- Fear
- Poor memory
- Moodiness

Medicinal
- Arthritis
- Bruises, sprains, or strains
- Burns (including sunburn)
- Wounds and scars
- Motion sickness
- Fatigue
- Respiratory conditions, such as colds, influenza, sore throat, asthma, and bronchitis
- Air purification
- Menstrual disorders
- Muscle aches and pains
- Fungal infections, such as athlete's foot and fungus nail
- Urinary tract infection
- Digestive disorders, such as constipation and indigestion

Skin care
- Dermatitis: eczema, acne
- Stretch marks
- Psoriasis
- Varicose veins
- Dry skin
- Cellulite
- Skin inflammation
- Wrinkles
- Wound healing
- Fungal infections

Note. From Natural Holistic Health, 2012

certification in aromatherapy should not randomly mix essential oils because some can be volatile. Specific uses include massage blends, baths, inhalation, hot and cold compresses, and fumigation. In massage therapy, blends of aromatic oils are used during massage. Massage therapy will be discussed in Chapter 9.

Bath Therapy

Bath therapy with essential oils can have profound effects on healing of skin disorders, alleviating muscle aches and pains, enhancing respiratory function, reducing stress levels, and increasing and supporting blood and lymph circulation. Essential oil baths, or aromatic bathing, facilitates healing on numerous levels, physiologically as well as psychologically.

In bath therapy, the water should be warm but not hot. The essential oils should be added to the bath just after or right before the individual gets into the water. The water should be swished around in order to disperse the concentration of essential oils. Note, if red blotches or irritation of the skin occurs while bathing, too much essential oil was added to the bath. In this case, a light cream without essential oils should be applied; the irritation should dissipate within one hour.

Aromatic baths with Epsom salts or sea salts are highly effective in aiding and supporting the body in detoxing and in wound healing. Epsom salts aid the elimination of waste material from the skin, reduce muscle aches and pains by aiding the elimination of uric acid build-up, and support and enhance the body's immune responses by stimulating lymph and blood circulation. The recommended amount is five to eight drops of essential oil per cup of Epsom salts.

Foot and hand baths can be utilized for the treatment of arthritis, athlete's foot, poor circulation, low energy, stress, nail fungus, and other skin disorders of the hands and feet. For an aromatherapy foot or hand bath, add five to seven drops of essential oil to a basin of warm or hot water and soak feet or hands for 10 to 15 minutes. One-half cup of Epsom salts can be added for an additional benefit.

Inhalation Therapy

Inhalation can be utilized for the treatment of various respiratory disorders as well as emotional states. It is most effective for treating respiration disorders involving nasal or chest congestion or an excess or deficiency of mucus (for example, sinusitis, bronchitis, hay fever, and postnasal drip). Various methods of inhalation therapy exist.

For *steam inhalation,* bring 2 cups of water to boil, reduce the heat, and let the water cool for 5 to 10 minutes. Then, add two to five drops of essential oil (or a combination of two to three essential oils). Inhale the vapors for 5 to 10 minutes. Place a towel over the head to increase the concentration. With steam inhalation, it is critical to keep the eyes closed to avoid irritation. Inhalation can be used two to three times per day.

Inhalation therapy can also be achieved using a handkerchief or a tissue. Place two to four drops of essential oil on the tissue or cloth. Hold the cloth in the palms and take two to three deep breaths through the nose several times per day. Another variation on this theme is to place two to four drops on a pillowcase during the night. This keeps the sinuses open throughout the night. For example, someone who is having trouble falling asleep can use eucalyptus and a drop of lavender to aid sleep.

Aerial Dispersion via Aerial Diffusers

Aerial dispersion via electric diffusers or nebulizers, is used for respiratory ailments, environmental air freshener, sedation or stimulation, emotional upset, and air purification for better quality and also for reduction airborne pathogens. Aerial dispersion is best utilized in short durations, and the recommended usage time is 15 minutes every 2 hours. The ionized microdroplets stay suspended in air for a while (NAHA, 2014b).

Christmas potpourri, clay candles, and electric pottery diffusers are other methods of aerial diffusion. Although these applications may not be considered medicinal, they do have therapeutic value. These types of diffusers are useful in the treatment of emotional upset and also provide a pleasant atmosphere. They are a very simple method of environmental fragrancing that can be used to enhance and beautify the home or office environment. A wide variety of clay diffusers are available in retail stores. Such diffusers include clay car diffusers, clay necklaces, glass necklaces, and small-room clay diffusers. These products are all useful in creating an aromatic environment to enhance emotional well-being.

Hot or Cold Compress Therapy

This method of application is best used in treating such conditions as muscular aches and pains, varicose veins, sprains, bruises, menstrual cramps, and respiratory congestion. It is also a wonderful way to relax after a long day at work. Use a cold compress for recent conditions and a hot compress for long-standing conditions or menstrual cramps. To prepare a compress, place five to seven drops of essential oil in 0.5 L of water. Swish the water around, and then place a washcloth or a piece of linen or cotton fabric into the water. Wring the fabric out and then place it on the area to be treated. Allow the compress to cool or heat, as appropriate, to body temperature and then remove it.

RELATED PROFESSIONAL ISSUES

Certification and Licensure

Although the cosmetic use of aromatherapy, such as aroma baths and aroma massage, does not require special consideration other than reading the manufacturer or store directions, the use of aromatherapy for therapeutic purposes must be guided by an expert practitioner. Essential oils can be used to make pastes, creams, gels, salves, compresses, and other aromatherapy applications. However, these procedures should only be carried out by trained and qualified aromatherapists. By learning more about the proper use of essential oils, either through a recognized school or through a qualified aromatherapy practitioner, one can open the door to a whole new world – one that is less dependent on conventional antibiotics and other overprescribed drugs (Buckle, 1997; Micozzi, 2001).

Currently, there are no regulatory agencies or bodies that oversee aromatherapy training courses or state or federal licensing of aromatherapists. However, a curriculum and standards exist. These have been developed by the NAHA and the American Holistic Nurses Association (AHNA) in the United States and by several international aromatherapy organizations. Certification is provided through educational programs that provide training in aromatherapy. Many schools and programs exist in different states and internationally. Courses vary from school to school and state to state. These various organizations and schools strive to maintain the appropriate and required standards set forth by the NAHA and AHNA. The NAHA aromatherapy curriculum and list of schools can be found at http://www.naha.org/education/standards.

Legal and Ethical Responsibilities

By learning more about the proper use of essential oils, either through recognized schools or through qualified aromatherapy practitioners, nurses can explore others ways of managing many of the preventable, acute and chronic conditions common in today's society. However, it is the nurse's professional, legal, and ethical responsibility to ensure appropriate training and documentation prior to recommending any essential oil use to a client.

Before purchasing and using essential oils at home or recommending their use to others, it is always best to seek the advice of a professional, qualified aromatherapy practitioner. Nurses should also take time to study the specifics of each essential oil. Although aromatherapy is not intended to replace conventional medicine or health care therapies, it can promote self-care, enabling individuals to take responsibility for their own health, and allow nature to do what it does best – balance and heal the body, mind, and spirit.

Client Safety Issues

Aromatherapy is extremely safe when used as recommended under the care of a qualified practitioner. However, it is important to remember that essential oils are very concentrated and could be volatile. Choosing the appropriate oil is as important as selecting the proper medication for any health problem. In addition, many essential oils are toxic. **Do not use too much of any essential oil.** It is a good idea to keep the eyes closed while inhaling these oils. This prevents fumes from irritating the eyes at close range and also helps build up imagery, which enhances the effects of essential oils.

Caution is recommended for patients who are pregnant or have asthma, high blood pressure, or epilepsy. People with allergies to any essential oil should not inhale that type of oil, and individuals with asthma must use caution with aromatherapy agents. Essential oils should also be used with caution with young children or babies. (See Table 3-5 for additional aromatherapy precautions.)

TABLE 3-5: AROMATHERAPY PRECAUTIONS

- Pregnant women should not use certain oils, such as camphor and hyssop.
- The first time a new essential oil blend is used, perform a patch test on the inside of the forearm to check for allergic reaction.
- Essential oils should be kept out of the reach of children.
- Some essential oils, such as rosemary, can raise blood pressure.
- Use synthetic aromatherapy products cautiously.
- Read essential oil labels carefully. Some oils that claim to be "natural" are fake, adulterated, or synthetic.
- Avoid products with artificial coloring, synthetic chemical additives, and added fragrances.
- Essential oils that can cause insomnia, such as mint oil, should not be used at night.

Oral consumption of essential oils is strongly discouraged unless the client is under the care and supervision of an experienced practitioner. If an essential oil comes in contact with the eyes or is accidentally spilled on the skin, rinse the eyes or wash the skin immediately with whole milk. Milk with some fat in it is best for reducing irritation and actually removing the oil. Oil or another vegetable oil can also be used for skin reactions that may result from essential oils, for example, a burning sensation in response to peppermint oil. If an essential oil is accidentally consumed, drink milk, eat soft bread, and go to the nearest poison control center for appropriate treatment (Ballard, O'Brien, Reichelt, & Perry, 2002).

CONCLUSION

Aromatherapy is as old as humanity itself. Although the Egyptians were the first true aromatherapists, the practice and use is worldwide. The practice is the use of essential oils from plants to balance, harmonize, and promote the health of the body, mind, and spirit. Aromatherapy is based on the idea that boosting the body's defense mechanism and immune system via touch and smell can promote and maintain health and restore energy balance.

Most essential oils have a variety of properties. Some act as antiseptic, antiviral, anti-inflammatory, analgesic, antidepressant, decongestant, or expectorant agents, whereas others have stimulating, uplifting, sedating, refreshing, calming, rejuvenating, toning, warming, cooling and relaxing effects. When used appropriately, their therapeutic effect for both medicinal and cosmetic reason are extremely safe.

ONLINE RESOURCES FOR AROMATHERAPY

Aromatherapy Holistic Online
  http://www.holistic-online.com
  Aromatherapy/hol_aroma.htm

Aromatherapy
  http://www.vitalspark.ca

Aromaweb
  http://www.aromaweb.com

Herbal Remedies
  http://www.herbalremedies.com

National Association of Aromatherapy
  http://www.naha.org

Aromatherapy
  http://www.aromatherapy.com

The Skeptic Dictionary
  http://skepdic.com/aroma.html

The International Center for Reiki Training
  http://www.reiki.org

West Coast Institute of Aromatherapy
  http://www.westcoastaromatherapy.com

EXAM QUESTIONS

CHAPTER 3
Questions 14–22

Note: Choose the one option that BEST answers each question.

14. The NAHA defines *aromatherapy* as the art and science of utilizing naturally extracted aromatic essences from

    a. animals.
    b. vitamins.
    c. plants.
    d. birds.

15. The French chemist Rene Maurice Gattefosse was the first person to transform the practice of aromatherapy from anecdotal science to today's well-recognized CAM therapy. Gattefosse coined the term *aromatherapy* in

    a. 1850.
    b. 1910.
    c. 1930.
    d. 1950.

16. The nursing theorist who used essential oils to enhance the healing environment was

    a. Jean Watson.
    b. Margaret Neuman.
    c. Florence Nightingale.
    d. Dorothy Orem.

17. Aromatherapy operates on the basic premise of the function of smell via the

    a. limbic nerves.
    b. olfactory nerve.
    c. olfactory system.
    d. acoustic system.

18. The method of extracting essential oils that uses steam or water is

    a. maceration.
    b. distillation.
    c. effleurage.
    d. expression.

19. The essential oil extraction method that is used exclusively to extract essential oils from citrus fruits is

    a. maceration.
    b. distillation.
    c. effleurage.
    d. expression.

20. During steam inhalation, it is critical to

    a. keep the eyes open.
    b. keep one eye open and the other closed.
    c. keep both eyes closed.
    d. close the eyes and the mouth.

21. The organizational body that set the current standards for the practice of aromatherapy is the

    a. American Nurses Association.
    b. National Association for Holistic Aromatherapy.
    c. Aromatherapy Association of America.
    d. World Health Organization.

31

continued on next page

22. The first time a new essential oil blend is used, it is important to perform a

    a. breathing test.

    b. blood test.

    c. urine test.

    (d.) patch test.

CHAPTER 4

HERBAL THERAPY

CHAPTER OBJECTIVE

Upon completion of this chapter, the learner will be able to describe the history, properties, and actions of herbal therapy and its uses as a holistic alternative and complementary therapy.

LEARNING OBJECTIVES

After studying this chapter, the learner will be able to:

1. Describe the history of herbal therapy.
2. Identify common herbs currently used in herbal therapy.
3. Differentiate herbal therapy from other similar therapeutics, such as aromatherapy, naturopathic medicine, and homeopathy.
4. List the benefits of herbal therapy as a holistic alternative and complementary therapy.
5. Identify at least ten of the most commonly used herbs and their adverse effects.
6. Discuss the nursing responsibilities and implications associated with herbal therapy use.
7. Identify various resources for information on the safe and effective use of herbal therapy.

INTRODUCTION

Herbal therapy has been used by man throughout time and has been handed down from generation to generation in many cultures as a form of folk medicine. It is the most widely used and oldest form of medicine in the world. Herbs are the original source of all medications

and, for many cultures, they continue to be the primary source of medicine. Herbs are also used for culinary and aromatic purposes.

Although herbal products have been used for centuries for healing, they can have negative effects and may interact with conventional drugs. Therefore, nurses must be informed about the actions, uses, recommended dosages, interactions, precautions, side effects, adverse effects, and nursing implications for every herb they administer or recommend to any client. That includes explaining the rationale to the client, monitoring the client for untoward effects, and educating the client about the need to read labels and understand safety precautions for each herb prior to ingestion. The purpose of this chapter, therefore, is to describe the history, uses, benefits, practical application, and nursing responsibilities associated with herbal therapy as a holistic alternative and complementary therapy.

DESCRIPTION OF HERBAL THERAPY

Herbal therapy, which is also known as *botanicals,* and *phytomedicine,* is the oldest therapy known to man. Herbs are considered dietary supplements. Parts of herbs used in herbal therapy include leaves, flowers, fruit, seeds, stems, bark, roots, and rhizomes. Herbal remedies are dispensed as liquids or powders and may be used in cooking and beverages or ingested in other forms. Herbalists are commonly known as *shamans* or *traditional healers* and can also make ointments and poultices out of herbs. Herbal therapy is fast becoming a mainstream natural, alternative, and complementary therapy. Some commonly used herbs with therapeutic value are echinacea (immune stimulant and anti-infection agent); garlic (antihypertensive and antibiotic); ginger (antinauseant and antispasmotic); ginseng root (increased stamina and decreased fatigue); kava kava (calming effect); and St. John's wort (anxiolytic and antidepressant).

Many definitions of herbal therapy exist. *Mosby's Medical, Nursing, and Allied Health Dictionary* (Anderson, Anderson, & Glanze, 2002) defines an *herb* as

1. a plant that is used for culinary and medicinal purposes
2. a plant with aerial parts that do not persist from one year to the next.

When used for therapeutic purposes, herbal therapy has some similarities to aromatherapy, naturopathic medicine, and homeopathic medicine. The basic differences between these therapeutic modalities are

- parts of the plant used
- method of extraction
- amount of the extract used
- how and when the therapy is used.

For example, aromatherapy deals specifically with the extraction and use of essential oils from plants. (See Chapter 3 for more information on aromatherapy.) In addition, herbal therapy is a key part of Chinese medicine, Indian ayurveda, and African healing practices. Some of these alternative and complementary therapies will be discussed in later chapters.

Herbal products are increasingly being used by the public for self-therapeutic and preventive purposes. In fact, the sale and use of herbal products for medicinal purposes in

the United States have reached a record high in recent years (Eisenberg et al., 1998; Lee, 1999; Pinn & Pallett, 2002). This renewed public interest in the use of herbs led Congress to pass the Dietary Supplement Health and Education Act (DSHEA) in 1994. The primary purpose of this act was to reclassify vitamins, minerals, and herbs as dietary supplements. This reclassification reduced the amount of control the U.S. Food and Drug Administration (FDA) has on monitoring and regulating the use of these products by the public. As a result, the FDA must prove that an herbal preparation is unsafe before the product can be forced off the market. This regulation, which no longer subjects herbs to the strict safety standards of conventional drugs, has made it possible for people other than herbalists, pharmacists, and physicians to be involved with the sale and recommendation of herbal therapies and preparations (NIH, 1994).

Until the 1950s, the FDA regulated herbs as drugs and most drugs used in conventional medicine originate from herbs. For example, the drug digitalis (cardiac glycosides), made from the foxglove plant, is used to treat congestive heart failure, and the drug aspirin, which derives from willow bark, is well known for its analgesic, anti-inflammatory, antipyretic, and anticoagulant-antiplatelet properties. Table 4-1 presents some drugs that originated from herbs and are still commonly used today. These drugs go through the full process of FDA review and approval.

HISTORY OF HERBAL THERAPY

The use of herbal products to treat illness dates back to the earliest records of mankind and is common to many cultures. Herbal therapy is used globally today. For example, herbal therapy, or phytomedicine (the science

TABLE 4-1: COMMON DRUGS THAT ORIGINATED FROM HERBS

Drug	Plant or Herb
Digitalis	Foxglove
Reserpine	Snakeroot or rauwolfia
Paclitaxel (Taxol)	Pacific yew
Aspirin	Willow bark
Atropine	Belladonna
Caffeine	Coffee shrub and cola nut
Emetine	Ipecac root
Ergotamine	Ergot alkaloid
Quinidine and quinine	Cinchona bark
Theophylline	Tea shrub

of botanical medicine), is prescribed by the majority of doctors in Germany, Asia, and many third-world countries. In Germany, government-provided health insurance even pays for herbal medicine (Holistic-online, n.d.-c).

Although the history of herbal therapy can be traced to Neanderthal times, in recent years, certain countries have begun to revolutionize the practice. In Germany, Belgium, Italy, Spain, the Netherlands, and certain Asian and African countries, herbs are used more consistently than in America (Flaherty et al., 2001; Lee, 1999; Pal & Shukla, 2003). In Germany, as in other European, Asian, and African countries, the history and use of herbs is well documented in many well-known monographs. For example, the German Commission E monographs (GCE monographs), also called the "Doctrine of Reasonable Certainty," which was formed in 1978, has been translated into English and is now widely used. Only recently did the United States publish its own comprehensive herbal list in the *Natural Medicine Comprehensive Database* (Jellin, Gregory, Batz, Hitchens, et al., 2000).

Until the 1950s in America, the federal government regulated herbs as drugs. However,

several landmarks in the history of the FDA regulation have resulted in changes in the use of herbal therapy (Eisenberg et al., 1998):

- 1938: The Federal Food, Drug, and Cosmetic (FFDC) Act required all new drugs, including herbs, to be proven safe before they were sold to the public.

- 1962: Kefauver-Harris Drug Amendments sought to amend the 1938 FFDC Act by requiring manufacturers for the first time to prove to the FDA a drug's effectiveness before selling it to the public. Many herbal manufacturers responded by marketing their product as dietary supplements. In response, the FDA considered these herbal products foods rather than drugs, and manufacturers were able to bypass this amendment.

- 1976: The Vitamins and Minerals Amendment was passed, prohibiting the FDA from limiting supplement potency or regulating supplements as drugs based solely on potency.

- 1990: The Nutrition Labeling and Education Act, which required that all packaged foods bear nutrition labels, included "herbs, or similar nutrition substances" in the definition of dietary supplements. Also, for the first time, the act permitted some health claims for certain foods and herbal products.

- 1994: DSHEA narrowly defined "dietary supplement" as a vitamin, a mineral, an herb or other botanical, an amino acid food, or a dietary substance for use by man to supplement the diet. Under the DSHEA, herbs can be labeled according to their effects on the structure and function of the body and the well-being achieved by consumers.

- 1999: The first Dietary Supplement Research Center was established in collaboration with the National Center for Complementary and Alternative Medicine.

- 2007: The FDA issued Good Manufacturing Practices (GMPs) for dietary supplements, which required manufacturers to guarantee the "identity, purity, strength, and composition" of their products. Other goals of the GMPs were to prevent inclusions of wrong ingredients or contaminants (i.e., pesticides, heavy metals, bacteria, etc.), to guarantee correct ingredient amounts, and to ensure proper packaging with truthful, nonmisleading labeling (National Institutes of Health [NIH], 2011). Also in 2007, manufacturers had to start reporting all serious dietary supplement related adverse events or illnesses to the FDA (Food and Drug Administration [FDA], 2014a) .
- 2014: FDA regulations *21 CFR part 111* (2007) remains in effect for all domestic and foreign companies that manufacture, package, label or hold dietary supplement for U.S. distribution and they must comply with the Dietary Supplement Current Good Manufacturing Practices (CGMPs) for quality control (FDA, 2013, 2014b)

Although dietary supplements do not have to be standardized in the United States, manufacturers are required to follow minimum quality standards. Standardization provides a measure of quality control that ensures all batches of a product are consistently uniform. Dietary supplements also do not have to be tested for efficacy or safety specifically, but the manufacturers and distributors of these products are responsible for ensuring their safety before they go to market. The FDA can authorize removal from market if they are found to be unsafe, adulterated, or if the claims on the products are false and misleading (FDA, 2014a; NIH, 2011).

These landmarks have political, social, and other implications on the history of herbal therapy use, which continues to increase globally.

HERBAL THERAPY PRACTICE

The holistic uses and benefits of herbal therapy cannot be understood without putting them in a cultural context. For instance, Africans, Asians, and Native Americans have used herbal therapy for thousands of years in combination with other therapies, such as music, meditation, dance, and prayers, to promote healing. Spirituality and herbs are inseparable in these cultures. For example, the process of making an herbal tea by an herbalist in Nigeria or a Native American is guided by a belief in God, who may also be called "Great Spirit," "Creator," or "One Who Oversees All Things." These traditional healers and herbalists focus their healing powers on creating a balance of harmony between the mind, body, and spirit (Cerrato, 1997; Huebscher & Shuler, 2003).

Herbal teas, which are medicinal beverages prepared by infusing the water-soluble extract of leaves, roots, barks, or other parts of an herb, are commonly used in many parts of the world. According to the World Health Organization (WHO), the use of herbal teas and baths is a common practice in many underdeveloped countries, where conventional drugs are not always available (WHO, 1998). The WHO, the American Holistic Nurses Association (AHNA), and researchers such as Goldman and Koren (2003); Lee (1999); and Allaire, Moos, and Wells (2000) recognize herbal therapy as a holistic therapy. In addition to tea infusions and baths, herbs can also be used as extracts, oils, salves, capsules, tablets, syrups, tinctures, juices, powders, decoctions, creams, lotions, and poultices.

Benefits of Herbal Therapy

Like drugs, herbs can be classified according to their physiological effects on the body. It should be noted, however, that based on the FDA classification and the 1994 DSHEA classification of herbs as dietary supplements, manufacturers cannot claim that an herb has medicinal properties unless the herb undergoes a rigorous approval process. Furthermore, manufacturers must ensure that labels are not misleading and that all labels bear a disclaimer indicating that the FDA has not reviewed the herb and that it is not intended to be used as a drug (NIH, 1994).

Physiologically, herbs can act as antispasmodics, diuretics, anti-inflammatory agents, vasodilators, sedatives, estrogen replacements or suppressants, antibacterials, antivirals, muscle relaxants, and antipyretic agents. Therefore, herbal remedies are used to treat physical illnesses such as asthma, diarrhea, coughs, colds, burns, digestive disorders, fevers, circulation problems, and infections. In some cultures, herbs may also be used for contraceptive purposes and for many female and male genitourinary issues (Allaire, Moos, & Wells, 2000; Goldman & Koren, 2003; Gozum & Unsal, 2004; Griffiths, 2000). Table 4-2 presents a list of commonly used herbs along with their uses and selected nursing implications.

RELATED PROFESSIONAL ISSUES

Certification and Licensure

Because the FDA generally does not classify herbs under the same category as drugs and because every culture has its own uses and names for the same herbs, there is a lack of standardization among herbal products. Although the debate about the efficacy of herbal therapy, the lack of standards, and the potential harm that herbs can cause continues, the public continues to increase its use of herbal products, as evidenced by an annual increase of billions of dollars in spending. According to

the American Botanical Council's 2013 report, herbal dietary supplement sales rose 5.5% in 2012, reaching an estimated 5.6 billion dollars (USD), the ninth year of consecutive growth (American Botanical Council, 2013).Therefore, to ensure public safety, regulations and standards are greatly needed in the United States to clarify the roles of the public and the various health care professionals currently involved in the sale, distribution, prescription, and recommendation of herbal products (Donaldson, 2002; Flanagan, 2001; Pal & Shukla, 2003).

Although many people believe that herbs should be treated as drugs, unlike drugs, there are no pressures by the U.S. government on the issue of who should or should not recommend these herbs. Naturopathic medicine, which includes the use of herbs, requires that individuals complete 2 years of university study and a 4-year program before they are allowed to practice. This is not true with herbal therapy, especially in many developing countries (Szelenyi & Brune, 2002). The AHNA provides nurses with a list of qualified practitioners and a list of courses or schools that promote and teach or focus on herbal medicine and other holistic therapies.

Legal and Ethical Responsibilities

Generally, the nursing role in herbal therapy involves education, administration, and monitoring. However, the majority of herbal products are available over the counter (OTC) and can be purchased by anyone. Despite this, it is important for nurses to understand the value of herbs in healing as well as the potential adverse effects and drug interactions. Nurses who are well trained and well informed can make recommendations on the use of herbs. However, it is the nurse's legal and ethical responsibility not only to be well informed about herbal therapy but also to be able to appropriately inform the client about herbs and

TABLE 4-2: COMMONLY USED HERBS AND BOTANICALS* (1 OF 2)

Herb/Botanical	Indications	Precautions
Alfalfa (*Medicago sativa*)	Allergies, arthritis, ulcers, indigestion, constipation	May cause bone marrow depression.
Aloe vera (*Aloe barbadenis*)	Wound healing, digestive aid, analgesic	Long-term use may cause arrhythmias, neuropathies, edema, and hematuria.
Black cohosh (rattle root, bugroot)	Antispasmodic, astringent, diuretic, premenstrual syndrome (PMS), infertility, vasodilation	Avoid use during pregnancy and lactation and in children.
Chamomile (*Matricaria recutita*)	Sleep aid, digestion, anti-inflammatory agent	May cause allergies and uterine relaxation.
Cranberry (*Vaccinium macrocarpon*)	Prophylactic for urinary tract infection (UTI)	Diabetics should take sugar-free cranberry. Can cause diarrhea with excess use.
Echinacea (*E. angustifolia* or *purpurea*)	Viral and fungal infections, cold, flu, for impaired immune function, wound healing	May cause fever or allergies. Contraindicated in progressive disease.
Ephedra (Ma Huang or *E. herba* or *sinensis*)	Energy stimulant, appetite suppressant, weight loss, allergies, asthma, coughs, colds	Banned by FDA in April 2004. See FDA caution.
Evening primrose (*Oenothera biennis*)	Natural estrogen promoter, PMS, diabetic neuropathy	May cause gastrointestinal (GI) upset, nausea, and headache.
Feverfew (*Tanacetum parthenium*)	Prophylaxis for migraine headaches, arthritis, menstrual problems	May cause mouth sores and rebound headache if discontinued abruptly.
Garlic (*Allium sativum*)	Diabetes, gastric and colorectal cancer, hypertension, high cholesterol, antiplatelet	May cause GI upset in high dosage and bleeding if taken with other anticoagulants.
Ginger (*Zingiber officinale*)	Anti-inflammatory, arthritis, antiemetic, morning sickness, motion sickness, vertigo	Considered safe by the FDA.
Ginkgo (*Ginkgo biloba*)	Increased blood flow to the central nervous system (CNS), mental alertness, antioxidant, Alzheimer's disease	Contraindicated in occlusive vascular disease. Can reduce clotting time.
Ginseng (*Panax quinquefolius*, *Panax schinseng*, or Chinese ginseng)	Fatigue, stress, impaired immune function, enhanced sexual function, increased energy levels	May cause euphoria, hypertension, insomnia, and vaginal bleeding.
Goldenseal (*Hydrastis canadensis*)	Skin and gum disease, indigestion, anti-inflammatory	Contraindicated in patients with diabetes, cardiac disease, glaucoma, or a history of cerebrovascular accident.
Kava kava (*Piper methysticum*)	CNS sedation for anxiety, insomnia, and skeletal muscle spasm; psychotic disorders	May cause unstable gait, GI upset, and liver damage.

TABLE 4-2: COMMONLY USED HERBS AND BOTANICALS* (2 OF 2)

Herb/Botanical	Indications	Precautions
Licorice (*Glycyrrhiza glabra*)	Antiulcer, antiviral, antitumor, anti-inflammatory, antibacterial, antidepressant, expectorant	May cause sodium retention. Use cautiously in patients with renal or cardiovascular disease.
Peppermint (*Mentha piperita*)	Antispasmodic, external analgesic, carminative for irritable bowel syndrome (IBS), indigestion, infant colic, nasal decongestant	None known.
Psyllium (*Plantago psyllium*)	Laxative; treatment of Crohn's disease, hemorrhoids, colitis, and IBS	None known.
Sage (*Salvia officinalis*)	For longevity, poultice, wound healing, decreased hot flashes	May cause nausea, vomiting and oral irritations.
Saw palmetto (*Serenoa repens*)	Benign prostatic hypertrophy	Does not reduce hyperplasia, only the symptoms of it.
St. John's wort (*Hypericum perforatum*)	Mild to moderate antidepressant, anxiety	May cause photosensitivity and possible monoamine oxidase inhibition.

*The majority of these herbs are contraindicated during pregnancy and lactation and in children.
(Jellin, Gregory, Batz, & Hitchens, 2000; Blumenthal, Goldberg, & Brinckmann, 2000)

their possible adverse effects. For example, the herb ephedra was a popular stimulant and appetite suppressant. However, this herb also contains ephedrine and pseudoephedrine, which can stimulate the respiratory system, increase heart rate and blood pressure, and cause heart failure, stroke, and death. Historically, the FDA cautioned clients with heart disease, hypertension, thyroid disease, diabetes, prostate hypertrophy, or glaucoma not to use this herb and, in April 2004, the FDA banned its use in the United States. See Table 4-3 for more herbs that should be avoided.

Nurses must be informed about the actions, uses, dosages, interactions, precautions, side effects, adverse effects, and nursing implications for every herb they administer or recommend to clients. This includes explaining the rationale for use to the client, monitoring the client for untoward effects, and instructing the client about the need to read labels and safety precautions for every herb prior to ingestion. According to Holt

(1996), professional responsibilities regarding herbal therapy extend beyond merely understanding what is now known about natural products (Flanagan, 2001; Kiefer, Shah, Gardiner, & Wechkin, 2001). However, more research is needed to better understand these products as the use by the public continues to increase (Popoola, 2003a). Table 4-4 provides some public education information that should be provided to anyone interested in using herbal products for therapeutic reasons.

Contraindications and Safety Issues

When advertising their dietary supplements, manufacturers are allowed to make three types of claims, without proof or evidence: health claims, structure/function claims, and nutrient content claims. These claims can link food/herbs to a disease or health-related conditions, or extol the product's health benefits. There are different requirements associated with each claim, i.e., claims about a product's efficacy must have supportive data. Claims about how a

TABLE 4-3: COMMON HERBS TO AVOID

Herbs	Use	Potential Adverse Effects and Cautions
Ephedra	stimulant, diet supplement	Increased heart rate, increased blood pressure, stroke.
Senna	laxative	Fainting, loss of bowel function, cardiac arrhythmias.
Comfrey root	wound healing	Liver and bladder cancer (proven in laboratory animals). Sold as tea. Several European countries restrict its use.
Lobelia	asthma	Brain damage, death. Acts like nicotine and is contra-indicated for persons with cardiovascular conditions. Also called *Indian tobacco.*
Yohimbe	aphrodisiac for men; treatment for erectile dysfunction	Use is inconclusive. Increased heart rate and blood pressure, dizziness, nervousness, headaches.
Vinca major	infection	Liver, kidney, and neurologic damage due to the content of toxic alkaloid-like vinblastine and vincristine.

(Jellin et al., 2000; Blumenthal et al., 2000)

TABLE 4-4: EDUCATION AND GENERAL PRECAUTIONS

- Consult with an herbalist or a qualified practitioner prior to using any product.
- Provide written information relating to a specific herb or therapy.
- Proactively question about the use of OTC herbs without labels.
- OTC herb labels should be read in detail prior to use.
- If a serious reaction occurs, a sample of the suspected product should be sent for chemical analysis.
- Serious reactions should be reported to the Food and Drug Administration's MedWatch program (800-332-1088).
- Package warnings should not be ignored.
- Keep herbs out of the reach of children.
- Do not take herbs if you are pregnant or nursing or attempting to become pregnant.
- Except for one or two types of herbs, do not give herbs to infants or young children.
- Users should not expect to be miraculously cured by herb..
- The word "natural" on an herb label does not automatically means that the product is natural or safe.
- Advise to stop using an herb immediately if any side effects occur.
- Herbal medicine should not be confused with homeopathy, naturopathy, or aromatherapy. (See the glossary for definitions of each term.)
- Dosage information should be referred to an expert in the field or an herbalist.

supplement affects the structure or function of the body must be followed by the words "This statement has not been evaluated by the U.S. Food and Drug Administration (FDA). This product is not intended to diagnose, treat, cure, or prevent any disease" (NIH, 2014b).

Some clients may think that because herbs are labeled natural, they do not have any adverse effects. Unfortunately, not all herbs are safe. Herbs are generally contraindicated for children under age 2 (Blumenthal, Goldberg, & Brinckmann, 2000; Lilley & Aucker, 2003).

In addition, some herbs are harmful if taken inappropriately and others can interact with commonly used drugs. Since there is little government oversight on herbal products, clients should be advised to consult with a qualified herbalist, a naturopathic doctor, and their health care providers. Barrios (1999), Donaldson (2002), Eisenberg et al. (1998), and Vender (2003) estimate that millions of adults are at risk for potential drug interactions. Table 4-5 lists some potential herb-drug interactions.

In the United States, the FDA has implemented a program called MedWatch to address the issue of public safety with regard to the use of drugs and other medical products, including herbs. Any health care professional or individual can call the toll-free number 800-332-1088 to report adverse effects of any herb.

CONCLUSION

Herbal therapy is the oldest therapy known to man. The practice has been handed down from generation to generation and from culture to cultures as folk medicine. Generally, an herb is a plant that is used for culinary and medicinal purposes. While herbal therapy has gone through many historical, social, and political changes, herbs were regulated as drugs by the federal government until the 1950s when it was classified as food or dietary supplement.

Like drugs, herbs can be classified according to their physiological effects on the body. However, manufacturers cannot claim that an herb has medicinal properties unless the herb undergoes a rigorous FDA approval process. In addition, manufacturers must ensure that the labels are not misleading as some herbs have severe side effects and contraindications, like any drugs.

ONLINE RESOURCES FOR HERBAL THERAPY

Alternative Medicine
    http://www.alternativemedicine.com

American Botanical Council
    http://www.herbalgram.org

American Herbal Pharmacopoeia
    http://www.herbal-ahp.org

American Holistic Nurses Association
    http://www.ahna.org

Center for Food Safety and Applied Nutrition
    http://www.cfsan.fda.gov

Focus on Alternative and Complementary
    Therapies (FACT)
    http://www.ex.ac.uk/FACT

HerbNET
    http://www.herbnet.com

Herb Research Foundation
    http://www.herbs.org

TABLE 4-5: POSSIBLE DRUG-HERB INTERACTIONS

Drug Classification	Herbal Interactions
Corticosteroids	Echinacea, astragalus, licorice
Cardiac glycosides: Digoxin	Hawthorn, Siberian ginseng, licorice
Hypoglycemics	Chromium
Iron	Feverfew, St. John's wort
Monoamine oxidase inhibitors	Ginseng, yohimbe, ephedra, St. John's wort, licorice
Anticonvulsants: phenobarbital and phenytoin	Evening primrose
Anticoagulants: Warfarin	Feverfew, garlic, ginger, ginkgo, ginseng

Holisticonline.com
   http://www.holistic-online.com

National Center for Complementary and
   Alternative Medicine
   http://www.nccam.nih.gov

National Institute of Health
   www.nih.gov

National Institutes of Health (NIH) –
   Clinical Trials
   http://clinicaltrials.gov/search/open/
   term=herbal+medicine

National Institutes of Health (NIH) –
   Herbal Medicine
   http://www.nlm.nih.gov/medlineplus/herbal-
   medicine.html#cat57

National Institute of Medical Herbalists
   http://www.nimh.org.uk

Natural Medicines Comprehensive Database
   http://www.naturaldatabase.com

EXAM QUESTIONS

CHAPTER 4
Questions 23–30

Note: Choose the one option that BEST answers each question.

23. Herbal therapy is the study of

    a. artificial food processing.

    b. essential oils used for spiritual and medicinal purposes.

    c. plants used for culinary and medicinal purposes.

    d. pharmacology for healing.

24. The FDA regulated herbs as drugs up until the

    a. 1990s.

    b. 1970s.

    c. 1960s.

    d. 1950s.

25. Under the DSHEA, herbs can be labeled according to their effects on the structure and function of the body and the well-being achieved by consumers; therefore, they are considered

    a. a complementary therapy.

    b. an alternative therapy.

    c. dietary supplements.

    d. a botanical therapy.

26. Cranberry is primarily used for

    a. UTIs.

    b. sinus headaches.

    c. digestive or stomach problems.

    d. energy stimulation and appetite suppression.

27. One herb that has been banned by the FDA because of its harmful effects to patients is

    a. St. John's wort.

    b. ephedra.

    c. saw palmetto.

    d. peppermint.

28. St. John's wort is indicated for and commonly used as an

    a. antiulcer agent.

    b. anti-inflammatory.

    c. antitumor agent.

    d. antidepressant.

29. Ginger is indicated for and commonly used as an

    a. antiulcer agent.

    b. anti-inflammatory.

    c. antitumor agent.

    d. antidepressant.

30. For public safety, the FDA has implemented a program that allows any health care professional or other person to call a toll-free number to report adverse effects from any herb. This program is called

    a. PharmacyWatch.

    b. NursingWatch.

    c. MedWatch.

    d. EducationWatch.

CHAPTER 5

REFLEXOLOGY

CHAPTER OBJECTIVE

Upon completion of this chapter, the learner will be able to describe the history and practice of reflexology and its uses as a holistic alternative and complementary therapy.

LEARNING OBJECTIVES

After studying this chapter, the learner will be able to:

1. Describe the history of reflexology.
2. Recognize the holistic characteristics of reflexology.
3. Differentiate between reflexology and massage.
4. List the benefits and uses of reflexology as a holistic alternative and complementary therapy.
5. Describe the practice of reflexology its related professional issues.

INTRODUCTION

Reflexology is the physical act of applying pressure to the feet and hands using thumb, finger, and hand techniques that do not utilize oils, creams, or lotions. These techniques produce physiological changes in the body that promote holistic healing, wellness, and body balance. This ancient practice is based on the premise that there are zones and reflex areas located on the feet and hands that correspond to other body parts. The feet and hands are viewed as maps or mirrors of the body. Each part of a foot or hand represents a certain part of the body. According to this theory, reflexes can communicate with organs, glands, and other parts of the body. In fact, each foot has more than 7,000 nerve endings that facilitate this communication process.

The purpose of this chapter is to discuss the history of and key issues related to the use of reflexology as a holistic alternative and complementary therapy. The chapter also describes practical application of the techniques and tips for practitioners. It should be noted that although reflexology is a relatively safe practice, it should not be used as a substitute for conventional medical care; rather, it should be used as a complementary therapy.

DESCRIPTION OF REFLEXOLOGY

The Reflexology Association of America (RAA) defines reflexology as "a non-invasive complementary practice involving the use of alternating pressure applied to reflexes within reflex maps of the body, located on the feet, hands and outer ears" (RAA, 2011).

Reflexology is an ancient therapy designed to bring wellness and balance back to the body by correcting imbalances caused by such factors as stress, ill health, pain, improper diet, environmental allergies, and anything else that causes a person to feel unwell or imbalanced.

Reflexology involves the use of the hands and fingers to apply gentle pressure to specific zones, or energy channels, of the feet and hands. These zones correlate with other parts of the body. For example, the toes correspond to the head; the ball of the foot, to the heart and lungs; and the heel, to the intestines (see Figure 5-1). Reflexologists believe that poor diet, stress, lack of exercise, illness, and other factors can cause congestion in the feet, resulting in deposits of crystalline-like lumps around the nerve endings. By using deep pressure with the fingers, reflexology therapists can break down these waste materials, so that they can be carried away in the bloodstream and excreted from the body. Some theorists also believe that reflexology allows the transference of energy via the meridian or energy points.

HISTORY OF REFLEXOLOGY

Although reflexology is currently receiving a lot of attention, the ideas behind this ancient therapeutic modality are not new. Although no one culture can be given sole credit for the development and practice of reflexology, evidence exists that the ancient practice dates back as far as 2300 B.C. in the Egyptian culture (International Institute of Reflexology, n.d.a). Reflexology can also be traced to ancient East Indian, Japanese, Arabic, Grecian, European, African, and Native American cultures (Avis, 1999; Huebscher & Shuler, 2003).

Modern reflexology has its roots in the early 20th century, when Dr. William Fitzgerald, an American physician, redeveloped the practice in 1913. Dr. Fitzgerald, who is known as the "Father of Modern Reflexology," believed that specific interactions occur between zones of the

FIGURE 5-1: HOLISTIC REFLEXOLOGY

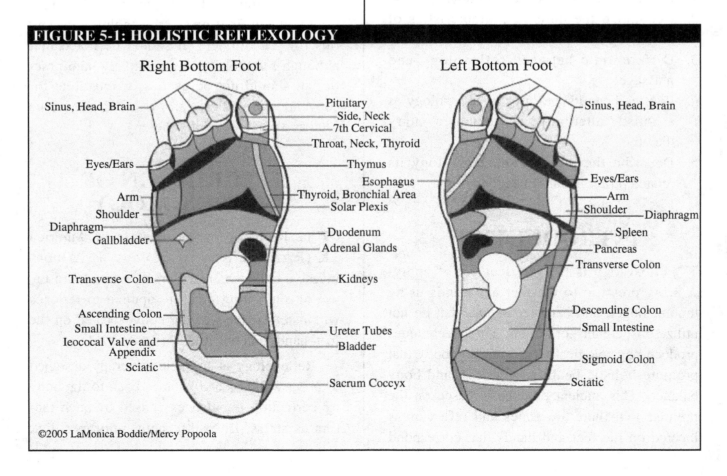

Right Bottom Foot — Left Bottom Foot

©2005 LaMonica Boddie/Mercy Popoola

hands and feet and the major organs of the body. He divided the body into ten equal and vertical zones. When stimulated, each zone affects all of the corresponding parts of the body for that zone. Later, in the 1920s, Dr. Joe Shelby joined in and continued the work of Dr. Fitzgerald. Dr. Shelby's contribution includes assisting with refining the division of the body into zones. Many years later, physiotherapist Eunice Ingham perfected the theory as it is known today, calling it the "Zone Theory of Foot Reflexology," and developed it into a usable therapy. She not only pinpointed which zones affected which parts of the body but also how.

Because many of the chronic health problems common in today's society are stress related, reflexology is fast becoming a well-recognized and commonly used alternative and complementary therapy, despite little scientific evidence that exists to support its efficacy. According to Avis (1999), reflexology is one of the most commonly used complementary and alternative therapies today. It is widely practiced, for example, in Europe, Denmark, Russia, and Germany for stress and disease management. In China, reflexology has been accepted by the central government as a means of preventing and curing diseases and preserving health. In Japan and Denmark, reflexology has been incorporated into the employer health programs of several large corporations, leading to savings in their annual sick leave benefits (Huebscher & Shuler, 2003; Smith, 2001).

REFLEXOLOGY PRACTICE

Principles of Reflexology

Reflexology is based on the theory that parts of the feet and hands correspond to and can therapeutically affect various other parts of the body. Reflexology works by reducing the amount of lactic acid in the feet and hands and breaking up calcium and other crystals that accumulate in the nerve endings and block the flow of energy (Huebscher & Shuler, 2003; Rankin-Box & Campbell, 2000; Smith, 2001). Although reflexology cannot be fully tested with the basic principles of physics, chemistry, and biology, it is a practice that is based on the holistic philosophy and has been perceived as a rational science with a strong ancestral base. In reflexology, when pressure is exerted on the hands or feet, a person becomes more relaxed and circulation improves. In addition, energy channels in the body are re-equilibrated, calcium deposits are loosened from tissues and joints, and natural endorphins are released to alter pain perception. Pain and stress relief occur, allowing the person to feel better and more relaxed.

Reflexology can be performed on oneself to an extent or done fully by another person. The equipment needed to perform reflexology is simple. A well-padded table, a chair or stool, and a quiet environment are usually all that is needed. However, reflexology can be modified to include other therapies, such as aromatherapy, nutrition therapy, relaxation and breathing exercises, herbal therapy, aquatic therapy, or music therapy, during and after the procedure.

Techniques

Various forms of reflexology exist, some of which have been around for centuries. Examples of techniques include the golf-ball technique, gentle-tough reflexology (Brygge et al., 2002; Mackey, 2001; Ricks, 1995), and the Ingham Method, or "Zone Theory." The Ingham Method is the most commonly used technique in the United States. It allows the practitioner to pinpoint the exact zone and location affected by the application of pressure. Different countries have slightly different variations of the techniques mentioned above.

In some cultures, reflexology is considered a type of massage therapy. However, reflexology involves much more than a simple foot massage. It involves foot or hand massage techniques that are intended to manipulate the thousands of nerve endings in these structures. Various massage and pressure techniques are used to relax tension and loosen toxins in the muscles and nerves, with the goal being to promote holistic healing and wellness. The procedures for performing foot massages and reflexology may be similar but, in reflexology, the focus is on application of pressure in the reflex zones in the feet and hands (see Figure 5-1).

Listed below are some recommendations for performing reflexology. These steps should be modified to meet the needs of the individual.

- Prior to beginning, ask the client about conditions that would contraindicate reflexology therapy (see Table 5-1). Advise client to seek advice from his or her physician if he or she has any concerns.

TABLE 5-1: ESSENTIAL TIPS TO REMEMBER BEFORE PERFORMING REFLEXOLOGY

- Always rule out a history of kidney stones, gallbladder stones, peripheral vascular disease, and vascular disease, including thrombosis and phlebitis.
- Avoid reflexology in pregnant women, except during labor.
- Aspiring or potential reflexologists should check with their state licensure boards prior to practicing.
- Reflexology is not a substitute for sound medical and nursing judgment or treatment.
- With certain health problem, use reflexology as a complementary therapy.
- For best results, use reflexology with other types of alternative and complementary therapies.

- Explain the procedure to the client and get his or her verbal or written permission to perform it. A physician's order is not required for a trained professional or certified practitioner.
- Create a quiet, healing environment, possibly with light aromatherapy.
- Position the client in a comfortable chair, such as a recliner, or on a treatment table or bed.
- Sit or stand in a comfortable position facing the client's soles or palms.
- Support the feet and hands as needed, especially for older clients.
- Assess the client's feet or hands for cuts, bruises, furuncles, or other abnormalities. If any abnormalities are present, do not perform reflexology. Gloves should be used when a break in the skin or a skin lesion is present.
- Encourage relaxation by assisting with breathing exercises.
- The use of oils, lotions, and creams before or during the application of reflexology is strongly discouraged because it blurs the lines between reflexology and massage and interferes with sensory feedback. However, the practitioner can rub a small amount of essential oils into his or her hands before practice to facilitate the process. Reflexology differs from massage because lotions, oils, creams, and essential oils are a critical part of massage therapy but not reflexology.
- Use the thumbs and fingers to apply gentle but firm pressure, and begin massaging one foot. Start at the toes use a kneading or wringing motion.
- Locate and continue to systematically apply pressure to each of the foot's reflex zones, paying special attention to the tender zone.
- Firmly hold the foot in one hand and press the thumb of the other hand on the sole, near the heel. Apply even pressure with the thumb and walk it forward. Continue pressing one spot at a time and moving forward to the toes.

- When you reach the toes, go back to the heel and trace another line from heel to toe.
- To finish, gently hold the foot for 30 seconds and have the client close his or her eyes to promote relaxation and closure.

Benefits of Reflexology

Reflexology has physiological and holistic benefits. According to the International Institute of Reflexology (n.d.-a), it is a holistic healing practice that has been found to have historically positive effects on the entire body. The ultimate goal of reflexology is to induce or maintain a state of balance and harmony in the body, mind, and spirit by blocking or interrupting unnecessary impulses that can result in illness and stress. Reducing stress and reestablishing the balance of energy are key benefits of reflexology.

Physiologically, reflexology improves nerve and blood supply and has the ability to promote healing. Another physiological benefit of reflexology is that, unlike pharmacological therapies, it has few, if any, side effects, contraindications, and interactions. It is a relatively safe practice that can be used for all ages. As a nonpharmacological therapeutic modality, it is used to promote blood circulation and can lead to improvement in many chronic physical and mental health conditions, such as fatigue and inflammatory diseases.

Like massage, reflexology is highly recognized and commonly used to reduce body tension, stress, and pain (massagetherapy.com, n.d.). Physicians, nurses, and massage and physical therapists who are trained in reflexology can use the practice as an alternative or complementary therapy to restore balance and promote relaxation. Reflexology can be used as an adjunctive, a complement, or an alternative to drug therapy. Some of the specific indications for reflexology use are listed in Table 5-2.

TABLE 5-2: SELECTED INDICATIONS FOR REFLEXOLOGY USE

Reflexology is indicated for
- stress
- muscle tension
- head, back, neck, and sinus pain
- earaches
- digestive or gastrointestinal problems, such as upset stomach, diarrhea, and constipation
- feet, knee, hip, and body pain
- hypertension
- migraines
- anxiety
- asthma.

Reflexology can also be used to
- relax women during childbirth
- reduce breast engorgement after delivery
- treat skin disorders such as eczema and acne
- relieve chronic inflammation, such as bursitis, laryngitis, arthritis, and tendinitis.

RELATED PROFESSIONAL ISSUES

Certification and Licensure

Recognizing that most reflexologists felt a desire to pursue the dream of a national association, the American Reflexology Certification Board (ARCB) hosted a conference in Denver, Colorado, in 1994, to explore such a possibility. Although the ARCB sponsored the conference, the ultimate outcome was in the hands of the participants. From this conference emerged a steering committee aimed at working toward the goal of establishing a national association. The 32-member committee worked for 1 year to bring the foundation for the association to a sufficient development to be presented for a vote at the conference. In St. Louis, a set of by-laws was adopted and an 11-member Board of Directors was elected on April 30, 1995, which officially founded the Reflexology Association of America (RAA). In 2003-2004, the RAA rewrote and passed new bylaws that changed its status from individual membership only, to a state-affiliated association with a 7-member Board of Directors. As of 2014, nineteen states had active affiliations with the RAA, each providing two delegates to serve on the RAA Delegate Assembly (RAA, 2014a). (Please see Table 5-3 for RAA State Affiliation List.)

TABLE 5-3: REFLEXOLOGY ASSOCIATION OF AMERICA (RAA) STATE MEMBERSHIP

2005:	Massachusetts
2006:	Colorado, Maryland, Maine, North Carolina, Rhode Island
2007:	Arizona, Ohio
2008:	Connecticut, Georgia, Missouri, New York
2009:	Iowa
2010:	Alaska
2012:	Florida, New Mexico, Oregon
2013:	Virginia
2014:	Wisconsin

Note: Reflexology Association of America (RAA), 2014a.

The RAA's Code of Ethics, along with its Standards of Practice, promote professional, ethical and confidential conduct within the field of reflexology; it has also differentiated itself from other holistic therapies by narrowing its scope of practice to specific techniques and areas of application (RAA, 2014b).

The process of obtaining reflexology licensure or certification varies from state to state. However, the RAA has formulated and reported the basic standards for obtaining certification in reflexology, which include the completion of a certain amount of hours in practice and testing. In some states, a massage license is required in order to practice reflexology. For the most part, however, any person in the medical field can become a reflexologist with properly documented training. No standard curriculum exists nationally that is mandated for certification and licensure.

Although members are not required to obtain national certification, the RAA encourages its members to achieve this goal, which demonstrates a higher level of competency. For organizations that wish to qualify as a certifying body, the RAA developed clear guidelines, within its policies and procedures, that followed the three criteria set forth by the National Commission for Certifying Agencies (NCAA) and the National Organization for Competency Assurance (NOCA). Both of these agencies are independent, non-profit, and non-governmental whose only purpose is to certify organizations that meet its standards.

In order to avoid any perceived or actual conflict of interest, the certifying body must be:

1. national in scope
2. non-profit (existing for the good of the profession, not for financial gain)
3. independent (not affiliated with any school, teacher, educational program, membership organization or other entity) (RAA, 2014c)

In 2013, the RAA Education Committee researched other certifying bodies in the U.S. in order to expand its certifying options, but as of 2014, the only agency that met RAA's criteria was the American Reflexology Certification Board (ARCB) (RAA, 2014c). To maintain a certification, the therapist must earn 12 hours of continuing education every two years post-certification.

For a more in-depth look into certificant requirements, please go to the American

Reflexology Certification Board website at http://arcb.net/cms/?page_id=223

According to Stone (2002) and the RAA, and in contrast with the United Kingdom, every state in the United States has its own licensing laws and regulations, determining which individuals have authorization to practice within a specialty. Although the RAA, a national organization, has clearly stated standards of practice, a code of ethics, and the scope of practice for reflexologists, the process of obtaining certification is still managed by each state. Therefore, the required course of study, process of certification, and legal responsibilities vary from state to state, making it mandatory for all aspiring reflexologists to check with the RAA and their board of certification prior to practicing on clients.

Treatment Precautions

Although reflexology can be beneficial, it should not be undertaken on anyone with a recent injury, wound on the foot or ankle or active gout until the individual is completely recovered. Other medical conditions that could pose a risk are diabetes, osteoarthritis on the foot or ankle, severe circulation problems affecting the lower extremities, certain cancers, heart disease, untreated hypertension, active infections, mental illness, pregnancy, gallstones and kidney stones. It is prudent to cover these areas during initial discussion and education, prior to starting therapy, and to encourage clients to talk to their doctors if they have concerns (Canyon Ranch, 2013).

Side Effects and Adverse Reactions

Clients may have different reactions to reflexology. Although rare, adverse reactions can occur. Because reactions are individualized, it is impossible to predict exactly how the body will react. According to the Danish

Reflexologists Association, some effects of reflexology therapy include:

- relaxation, tiredness, or deep sleep
- changes in bowel movements
- nose and throat secretions
- mood changes.

However, these reactions should be viewed as signs that the treatment is working and should not be viewed as adverse reactions (Stephenson & Dalton, 2003).

"Healing crisis" is a term that is associated with a number of complementary and alternative therapies, including reflexology. In reflexology, this crisis refers to a collection of symptoms that may occur, although rare, after reflexology. Manifestations may include fever, rash, diaphoresis, diarrhea, and nausea. These rare symptoms have been attributed to the release of toxins and actually serve as proof that the treatment is working. These symptoms usually go away within 1 day, and clients should be encouraged to see their physicians if the conditions persist.

CONCLUSION

Reflexology is an ancient practice that is based on the premise that there are zones, energy channels, and reflex areas located on the feet and hands that correspond to other body parts. Reflexology is a holistic healing practice of applying pressure to the feet and hands using thumb, finger, and hand techniques with the ultimate goal of inducing or maintaining a state of balance and harmony by blocking and interrupting unnecessary impulses that can result in illness and stress. Like massage therapy, reflexology is commonly used to reduce tension, stress, and pain with little or no side effects.

ONLINE RESOURCES FOR REFLEXOLOGY

Association of Reflexologists
   http://www.aor.org.uk

Home of Reflexology
   http://www.reflexology.org

The Universal healing Sanctuary
   http://www.reikihealing.co.za

Reflexology Research
   http://www.reflexology-research.com

EXAM QUESTIONS

CHAPTER 5
Questions 31–35

Note: Choose the one option that BEST answers each question.

31. One reflexology technique is the use of

    a. an instrument to apply pressure to the client's body.

    b. an ultrasound to apply gentle pressure to specific points on the client's feet and hands.

    c. the thumb and fingers to apply gentle pressure to specific points on the client's feet and hands.

    d. the fingers and the heels to apply gentle pressure to specific points on the client's feet and hands.

32. The earliest documentation of reflexology was recorded in Egypt in

    a. 2003 B.C.

    b. 2300 B.C.

    c. 2030 A.D.

    d. 2033 B.C.

33. One difference between reflexology and massage is that in reflexology

    a. the use of oils, lotions, and creams is strongly recommended.

    b. the use of oils, lotions, and creams is strongly discouraged.

    c. the RAA recommends always using a small amount of essential oils on the hands.

    d. the use of herbal cleansing agents and lotion ONLY are strongly recommended.

34. Despite a lack of scientific evidence to show that reflexology works, reflexology is highly recognized and commonly used to

    a. reduce body tension, stress, and pain.

    b. treat sinus headaches.

    c. treat digestive or stomach problems.

    d. relieve earaches.

35. Generally, the use of other types of alternative and complementary therapies in conjunction with reflexology is

    a. recommended with caution.

    b. highly recommended.

    c. not recommended.

    d. recommended after checking with the client's primary physician.

CHAPTER 6

AQUATIC THERAPY

CHAPTER OBJECTIVE

Upon completion of this chapter, the learner will be able to discuss the practice of aquatic therapy and its uses as a holistic alternative and complementary therapy.

LEARNING OBJECTIVES

After studying this chapter, the learner will be able to:

1. Describe the history of aquatic therapy.
2. List the properties of water that make aquatic therapy therapeutic.
3. Identify at least five of the most common methods of applying aquatic therapy.
4. Discuss one specific form of aquatic therapy
5. List the physiological and psychological benefits of aquatic therapy as a holistic alternative and complementary therapy.
6. Identify practical precautions that need to be taken when using aquatic therapy.
7. Discuss the nursing responsibilities and implications associated with the use of aquatic therapy.

INTRODUCTION

Aquatic therapy entails a purposeful progression of skills focusing on psychosocial, cognitive, leisure, and motor performance using the properties of water to enhance these experiences. Aquatic therapy is also commonly known as *hydrotherapy, water therapy,* and *aqua therapy. Hydrotherapy* specifically refers to the use of water by external application either for its pressure effect or as a means of applying energy to body tissue. One common use of aquatic therapy by health care professionals is for wound management; specifically, whirlpool baths are used to clean, disinfect, and granulate wounds; promote healing; and decrease pain (Hoffman et al., 2004; Peterson, 2001; Popoola, 2003b).

Aquatic therapy methods have been used for centuries by many religions and cultures for the treatment of disease and injury as well as for relaxation, stress reduction, anxiety, and acute and chronic pain management. For example, the ancient Greeks and Romans often took therapeutic baths for both social and therapeutic purposes.

In aquatic therapy, various forms of water, such as ice, liquid, and vapor are used internally or externally to promote healing. Hydrothermal aquatic therapy such as hot or cold baths, saunas, and wraps, also include the temperature effects of water to treat certain diseases. Aquatic therapy is an intervention that can be used to increase an individual's physical, social, cognitive, and spiritual domains. It is frequently used in spa therapy and in rehabilitation centers. This chapter discusses the practice of aquatic therapy and relates its uses as a holistic alternative and complementary therapy.

DESCRIPTION OF AQUATIC THERAPY

The skin is the largest organ of the body. The skin provides a very effective protection against invasive bacteria and other foreign matters. Aquatic therapy can be used to train the skin to more efficiently regulate warmth and circulation. It can stimulate the immune system, help increase the body's white blood cell count, aid the body in purging itself of accumulated toxins, and produce a state of general relaxation that can be essential to the healing process (Dossey, Keegan, & Guzzetta, 2000; Peterson, 2001; Prins & Cutner, 1999). It can also be effective in removing many toxins, parasites, bacteria, and viruses that can cause disease (Emmerson, 2001; Ridgway & Tedder, 1996).

According to Keegan (2003), aquatic therapy is one of the most widely used, evidence-based alternative and complementary therapies. Keegan (2003) describes aquatic therapy as some form of water used to augment healing. For example, regular swimming in cold water increases the body's resistance to bacterial and viral infections. Participating in water therapy at a spa for rehabilitation or leisure can generally improve health, help maintain a sense of well-being, and prevent tension and stress. Keegan (2003) notes that aquatic therapy can be used with other natural, alternative, and complementary therapies (NAC), such as aromatherapy, music therapy, and massage therapy, to manage stress and anxiety.

In addition to stress and anxiety management, aquatic therapy can be very useful in managing various physiological problems. For example, it can be used as a nonpharmacological pain-relief method to manage labor pain during deliveries (Benfield, 2002; Benfield, Herman, Katz, Wilson, & Davis, 2001; Prins & Cutner, 1999). According to Prins and Cutner

(1999), aquatic therapy is a safe, effective, and alternative intervention that can be used to help low-risk women cope with labor. Studies have shown the therapeutic benefits of this practice to expecting mothers include increased relaxation, increased satisfaction, increased cervical dilation, lower blood pressure, and increased diuresis with no increased risk of infection (Benfield, 2002; Peterson, 2001).

According to Benfield (2002), the use of water during labor or immersion during delivery, which is sometimes called "maternal bathing," can also rapidly relieve pain and anxiety. Although many studies support the efficacious use of aquatic therapy in labor, Benfield's (2002) study shows that no clear evidence exists to indicate that this therapy increases fetal descent, reduces uterine dyskinesia, shortens labor, or decreases the incidence of operative delivery or hemorrhage.

HISTORY OF AQUATIC THERAPY

Aquatic therapy has been around for centuries. Records of its use have been found in historical documents that date back as early as the 5th century B.C. In the river valleys of Mesopotamia, Egypt, India, China, and almost all cultures with access to water, soaking in bathtubs, rivers, oceans, pools, and spas is used for social and spiritual purposes (Becker & Cole, 1997). Healing water rituals were also used by ancient Greek, Hebrew, Roman, Christian, and Islamic cultures in order to cleanse the earthly body of disease and the spiritual body of sin. During and after World Wars I and II, the use of water increased and expanded to include exercise and maintenance or restoration of health, especially in the United States (Becker & Cole, 1997).

Aquatic therapy methods have been used for centuries by many religions and cultures for the treatment of disease and injury as well as for relaxation, stress reduction, anxiety, and acute and chronic pain management. For example, the ancient Greeks and Romans often took therapeutic baths for both social and therapeutic purposes. In addition, water is an important ingredient in some traditional healing practices, such as those of the Chinese, Egyptians, and Native Americans. According to Tella (1999) the physical and psychological benefits of swimming have long been established.

One well-known form of aquatic therapy is Watsu, or aquatic shiatsu, which is commonly used in rehabilitation centers. According to Osborn (2003) and the School of Shiatsu and Massage (2003), Watsu began in 1980 at the Harbin Hot Springs in Northern California, where Harold Dull brought his knowledge of Zen Shiatsu into a warm pool. Dull discovered that the effects of Zen Shiatsu could be amplified by stretching someone while he or she floated in warm water. Shiatsu is a type of holistic massage therapy that has a long traditional history in Asian cultures. According to Bright (2002), shiatsu is a type of healing bodywork that originated in China, India, Japan, Korea, and Thailand. Watsu and other specific types of aquatic therapy will be discussed later in this chapter.

AQUATIC THERAPY PRACTICE

Principles of Aquatic Therapy

Water has many properties that enhance its ability to create an environment that increases the overall quality of life. These properties include density and specific gravity, buoyancy factor, hydrostatic pressure, refraction and reflection factor, viscosity, stream flow, and turbulence.

Density is defined as mass per unit volume. **Specific gravity** is the relative density, or the ratio of the density of a body to the density of water. The specific gravity of water is 1. The specific gravity for a female is 0.75 and for a male is 0.95. Lungs deflate at a specific gravity of 1.05 to 1.08. This explains why people can float in water and can swim longer with their heads above water.

Buoyancy factor is the force of gravity that results in a feeling of weightlessness when immersed in water. Buoyancy factor decreases weight-bearing and joint compression forces, decreases the effort required with slow movements against gravity, and increases functional ability (Dattilo, 2000; Prins & Cutner, 1999).

Hydrostatic pressure is the pressure exerted by molecules upon an immersed body. The fluid pressure is equal at a given depth. Due to this property, swelling decreases with increased pressure, offsetting the tendency of blood to pool in extremities and helping to build the muscles of inspiration and exhalation. This also has a diuretic effect by increasing the amount of residual urine output.

Viscosity refers to the amount of cohesion molecules have to other matter. This property provides **resistance** with increased speed, which improves strength (Peterson, 2001; Prins & Cutner, 1999).

Turbulence refers to uneven patterns of water movement that can establish patterns of low-pressure areas following in the wake of an object moving through a fluid.

These water properties can be used to pull a body through the water by assisting the participant in swimming, ambulating, or walking (Ruoti, Morris, & Cole, 1997; Dattilo, 2000).

Therapeutic Properties

The healing properties of aquatic therapy are based on water's mechanical and thermal effects. Aquatic therapy, specifically hydrothermal therapy, exploits the body's reactions to hot and cold stimuli, the protracted application of heat, water pressure, and the sensations water gives. Nerves carry impulses felt at the skin deeper into the body, where they are instrumental in stimulating the immune system, influencing the production of stress hormones, invigorating circulation and digestion, encouraging blood flow, and lessening pain sensitivity.

Generally, heat quiets and soothes the body, slowing down the activity of internal organs. In contrast, cold stimulates and invigorates, increasing internal activity. For example, if a person is experiencing tense muscles and anxiety from stress, a hot shower or bath is always effective. For feelings of tiredness and stress, a warm shower or bath followed by a short, invigorating cold shower can help stimulate the body and mind.

When we submerge our bodies in a bath, a pool, or a whirlpool, we experience a kind of weightlessness. Our body is relieved from the constant pull of gravity. Water also has a hydrostatic effect and massage-like feeling as it gently kneads the body. Water in motion stimulates touch receptors on the skin, boosting blood circulation and releasing tight muscles. Some types of aquatic therapy, such as Watsu, are used to promote holistic healing and balance through the manipulation and balance of the life forces called *chi* (ki) and *prana*. Others, such as whirlpool baths, are used for wound healing and for promoting circulation.

Methods of Applying Aquatic Therapy

Dozens of methods of applying aquatic therapy now exist. A number of techniques are available under the general heading of "hydrotherapy." These include baths and showers, swimming, neutral baths, sitz baths, footbaths, cold mitten friction rubs, steam inhalation, hot compresses, cold compresses, cold and heat rubbing, douches, body wraps, wet sheet packs, and whirlpool baths (Holistic-online.com, n.d.-d; Ruoti, Morris, & Cole, 1997; Saeki, 2000). Some of these methods will be presented in this section.

Saunas and Steam Baths

Saunas and steam baths produce similar effects. Sauna is the use of a hot, dry, wood-lined room for relaxing while sitting or lying down and it encourages cleasing through perspiration by opening the pores and eliminating toxins through sweat. Steam bath, the wet version of sauna, is used also to promote perspiration and remove body toxins. Steam baths are not only relaxing, they are also cleansing, change body temperature, and promote blood flow. The decision to take one rather than the other is guided by personal preference. In a sauna, the heat acts more quickly to eliminate toxins through the skin, although some consider the moist air of a steam bath more satisfying to the respiratory system. Saunas are deeply relaxing and are a great way to melt away stress. Sauna baths stimulate blood flow, increase heart rate, have an immune-modulating effect, promote hormone production, encourage mucus secretion in the respiratory system, open the airways, reduce resistance to respiration, promote relaxation, and can improve mental outlook.

Full and Partial Immersion Baths

Immersion baths are types of baths in which the entire body, or only parts of the body, are submerged in water. Various substances can be added to warm water and rising temperature baths. Herbs are commonly used. (Herbal bath therapy was discussed in Chapter 4 and will also be addressed later in this section.) These bath therapies can be applied to different parts of the body, such as the hip, arm, thigh, and forehead. Two examples of immersion baths are the cold footbath and the sitz bath.

In a cold footbath, the feet are placed into a footbath filled to calf depth with cold water. Participants are encouraged to stop when a cold stimulus is felt or when the water is no longer perceived as being cold.

A sitz bath is a type of bath in which the hip, rectal, or perineal areas are immersed in water to decrease swelling, inflammation, and pain. A sitz bath is usually administered as cold, rising temperature or in warm bath. Parts of the body not immersed in water should be covered. Cold or warm sitz baths are effective for hemorrhoids or inflammation of the anus, difficulty voiding, irritable bladder, inflammation or infection of the prostate, and preparation for pregnancy or pain relief after vaginal delivery.

Wraps

A wrap is primarily used as a supportive measure for treating fever and local inflammation. The person receiving treatment should first adopt a relaxed position. Next, a linen cloth moistened with cold water (warm water for conditions such as respiratory diseases) and then well wrung is tightly wrapped around the appropriate part of the body, but not so tightly that it causes constriction. A dry cotton or linen cloth is then wrapped over the moist cloth. The patient is usually then wrapped in a blanket or another cloth and rests for up to 60 minutes. If the wrap is cool after a quarter of an hour, heat should be applied in the form of a hot water bottle or by giving warm tea. The wrap should be removed immediately if the person complains of feeling unwell or cold. Wraps are useful for sore throat (neck wrap), bronchitis and lung disease (chest wrap), pelvic infection, hemorrhoids, prostate problems (hip wrap), arthritis

(joint wrap), phlebitis from intravenous fluid infection, and edema (calf and arm wrap).

Warm and Cold Packs

In warm packs, a wrapping cloth is soaked in a hot infusion or decoction of herbs, wrung out and wrapped around the patient's specific body parts. Alternatively, the wrap may receive a coating of hot mud mustard flour. It is useful for treating painful chronic diseases, such as arthrosis and cystitis, and for stimulating blood flow.

In cold packs, ice or cooled cataplasm is spread onto a wrapping cloth and then placed on the affected part of the body. Crushed ice in a plastic bag may also be repeatedly applied for 1 minute, removed for 4 minutes, and then reapplied. Cold packs are useful for various joint inflammations, sprains and strains, pleurisy, and headaches.

Herbal Baths

Herbal baths can be particularly soothing when a person is experiencing stress. There are several ways to prepare an herbal bath, for example, in a tub or basin, as a shower, as a decoction into bath water, and as a wrap of herbs in a washcloth. Herbal baths involve soaking in a tub for at least 20 minutes or rubbing an herbal washcloth over the body. It is important to cover the drain with a thin mesh screen to prevent the herbs from clogging the pipes. Certain herbs are particularly effective for creating soothing baths, including valerian, lavender, linden, chamomile, hops, burdock root, yarrow, and passionflower. It is important to follow expert directions in the preparation of herbal baths and to mix herbs according to expert recommendations or those found on the manufacturer's label.

Watsu: A Form of Aquatic Therapy

There are several different forms of aquatic therapy. Among these are Watsu, the Bad Ragaz Ring Method, Halliwick, Ai Chi, the Dolan

Method, and aqua jogging. Aqua jogging is commonly used to maintain cardiovascular fitness and strength (Lutz, 1999; Michalsen et al., 2003; Peterson, 2001).

As previously mentioned, Watsu, or aquatic shiatsu, is a form of aquatic therapy that involves applying the stretches and moves of the Zen Shiatsu in warm water. Zen Shiatsu incorporates stretches that release blockages along the meridians (channels through which chi, or lifeforce, flows). In Watsu, the client floats in warm water, lessening resistance in the limbs. Watsu movements include rocking and stretching the whole body while supporting the joints. According to Osborn (2003) and Ruoti, Morris, and Cole (1997), Watsu lessens the resistance when isolating a limb, and the warmth and buoyancy of water are ideal for freeing the spine. It helps to decrease muscle tension, increase range of motion (ROM), facilitate deep breathing, decrease pain and stress, and improve body awareness. It is also often used in rehabilitation centers to treat traumatic injuries, such as brain and spinal cord injuries; orthopedic disorders; congenital birth defects, including spina bifida and autism; and other neurological disorders in children and adults.

According to Harold Dull (2004), who developed Watsu in the 1980s, the term means "body in water" or "freeing the body in water." Watsu aquatic therapy is a sequencing of gentle movements and stretching, as one is held or supported in warm water. This supportive movement can relax and nurture the whole body. This kind of supportive movement is impossible on land.

In Watsu, Shiatsu techniques are often used. Shiatsu, meaning "finger pressure," was developed in Japan but originated from the use of the chi, ki, and prana forces, which can be traced to traditional Chinese medicine. Zen Shiatsu is the most common type of Shiatsu. Watsu, however, combines the elements of massage, shiatsu, and movement therapy in warm water. Watsu also creates a deep connection through the kind of holding or cradling that being in water encourages. According to Ruoti, Morris, and Cole (1997), Watsu aquatic therapy has a more intimate approach than other therapies. Although clients may initially tense, they end up relaxed, with increased comfort and reduced pain.

Benefits of Aquatic Therapy

When used in therapy, the properties of water provide physical and psychological benefits to people with and without disabilities. Various case reports, observational studies, and controlled studies have provided some evidence of the success of aquatic therapy (Broach, Groff, & Dattillo, 1997; McCaffrey, 2000; Osborne, 2003).

Aquatic therapy has been proven to be effective in invigorating and toning up the body, and promoting blood flow. It can also be used in health promotion, such as for prevention of the common cold. In addition, it has been used to treat and manage:

- problems with circulation
- respiratory infections
- pain caused by pulled back muscles, sciatica, chronic rheumatoid arthritis, bronchial asthma, unstable hypertension, and severely disturbed peripheral blood circulation
- varicose veins
- edema
- headaches
- low blood pressure
- circulatory problems
- sleeplessness

(Holistic-online.com, n.d.-d).

Physiological Benefits

Aquatic therapy is an approach to healing that, according to Osborn (2003), can be used as an alternative to pharmacological treatment.

It is useful for decreasing pain, preventing bone loss, increasing strength and endurance, improving pulmonary function, returning function to clients with spinal cord injuries, and improving ROM. Increased physical functioning can lead to overall health benefits (Broach & Dattilo, 1996). Aquatic therapy is commonly used as an alternative therapy in the rehabilitation of individuals with disabilities. Aquatic swimming therapy programs for adults with spinal cord injuries have been studied for their physical benefits. For example, Broach, Groff, and Dattilo (1997) found that aquatic therapy improved the endurance of adults with spinal cord injuries.

Aquatic therapy is also used to tone the body, stimulate digestion, improve circulation, and boost the immune system. Water seems to have the ability to get rid of stress and rejuvenate the body. It affects the skin and muscles. It calms the lungs, heart, stomach, and endocrine system by stimulating nerve reflexes of the spinal cord. Table 6-1 lists some general physiological benefits of aquatic therapy.

Psychological Benefits

Aquatic or hydrotherapy is an example of a holistic NAC therapy (American Holistic Nurses Association [AHNA], 2014; Dossey, 2001). As a complementary therapy, aquatic therapy is useful in helping to eliminate toxic material from the body by encouraging sweating and cleaning. In order to reach a point of holistic living, an individual must be happy with his or her inner self. Aquatic therapy improves psychological functioning of individuals with and without disabilities. Specifically, it improves body image, decreases depression, enhances mood, and promotes self-determination and self-motivation. A significant reduction in anger, confusion, and tension has also been reported by people in aquatic therapy groups (AHNA,

TABLE 6-1: PHYSIOLOGICAL BENEFITS OF AQUATIC THERAPY

Decreases/prevents
- muscle contractions
- spasticity
- fatigue
- respiratory complaints
- swelling

Improves/increases
- strength
- ROM
- gait
- circulation
- oral and facial control
- coordination
- endurance
- healing of tissues
- independence in functional activity

2000). Aquatic therapy can also help alleviate tension, nervousness, and other symptoms that accompany anxiety attacks.

Warm baths with or without herbs can help soothe anxious states of mind and can be used for personal comfort, relaxation, and enjoyment. According to Sova (2004), water plays an important part in rest and relaxation. Once relaxed, individuals can focus on the issues or conflicts that are causing their anxiety. For any individual feeling anxious or irritated, a neutral bath with the right temperature and with the body submerged for at least 20 minutes has a balancing and soothing effect. A relaxing blend of essential oils, such as lavender, geranium, and bergamot in sweet almond oil or peach kernel oil, may be used in a bath at times of great stress and anxiety to increase the effects of aquatic therapy. When combined with other complementary therapies, such as music, baths can further relieve anxiety. In addition, hot moist compresses applied to the spine, hot foot baths, and hot water bottles placed on the feet can also be beneficial in relieving anxiety and stress.

It should be noted that aquatic therapy cannot cure anxiety disorders and is not a substitute for conventional medicine or treatment.

RELATED PROFESSIONAL ISSUES

Certification and Licensure

According to the Harbin School of Healing Arts in California, a private institution, originally owned by Harold Dull, the founder of Watsu®, anyone can become qualified and certified to perform aquatic body work or Watsu aquatic therapy by undergoing a program with a set number of training hours. There are several stages and many hours involved in Watsu training, with each stage teaching presence, flow, form, adaption, and creativity which are learned continuously throughout life. Rather than just being a step, each becomes a platform that supports and sustains the next (Harbin School of Healing Arts, 2014).

To obtain licensure, certification, and registration, it is important to first check with state, city, and county ordinances for licensing and bodywork training requirements in order to set up a practice. Nurses also have a legal and ethical responsibility to check the authenticity of any school they plan to attend before training to become an aquatic therapist (Harbin School of Healing Arts, 2014; Worldwide Aquatic Bodywork Association [WABA], 2014).

Aquatic therapy has come a long way. It is used by doctors, nurses, physical therapists (PTs), PT assistants, nursing assistants, and even patients for physical fitness and for healing purposes. Generally, nurses are not involved with full-body aquatic therapy

or the use of aquatic therapy for rehabilitation. Aquatic therapy is widely used in sports medicine and in rehabilitation centers by PTs and trained or certified nonlicensed providers, such as PT or nursing assistants (Wykle, 2003; Benfield, 2002). However, just like the general public, nurses can be involved in the recreational and stress-reduction uses of aquatic therapy for maintaining physical fitness, such as aquatic aerobics. According to Saeki (2000), foot bathing is also a frequently performed nursing practice. In fact, it was an important part of morning and evening care in the early days of nursing. Today, however, footbaths are rarely incorporated into morning or evening care. Nurses need to revisit the use of aquatic therapy such as footbaths which, according to the AHNA, is not only an alternative and complementary therapeutic modality but is a practice within the scope of nursing.

Water Precautions from the CDC and WHO

According to the Centers for Disease Control (CDC) and WHO, water is used in many areas of health care and it is essential for health and well-being. However, it is appropriate to note that when using aquatic therapy internally or externally for therapy, caution should be taken to maintain the hygienic quality of the water and the environment. According to the WHO (2014a), Wykle (2003), Benkel et al. (2000), and Simon (2004), potential problems of aquatic therapy could include water-borne infections, such as parasites and environmental infections.

Safety precautions are paramount when dealing with water therapy. Injuries, drownings and infections, such as, legionellosis, folliculitis, meningitis, otitis externa, and urinary tract infections are potential health hazards (Benkel et al., 2000; Simon, 2004). Drowning ranks fifth among the leading causes of unintentional injury death in the United States (CDC, 2014a). In 2007, The Virginia Graeme Baker Pool & Spa Safety Act (P&SS Act) was enacted by Congress and signed into law. It was designed "to prevent the tragic and hidden hazard of drain entrapments and eviscerations in pools and spas" (U.S. Consumer Product Safety Commission [CPSC], 2008).

Table 6-2 provides some key points to remember about using aquatic therapy and Figure 6-1 presents aquatic therapy as a holistic therapy.

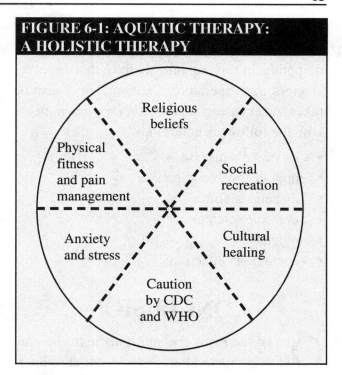

FIGURE 6-1: AQUATIC THERAPY: A HOLISTIC THERAPY

Religious beliefs

Physical fitness and pain management

Social recreation

Anxiety and stress

Cultural healing

Caution by CDC and WHO

TABLE 6-2: KEY POINTS REGARDING AQUATIC THERAPY USE

- According to CDC (2014a) in the United States, drownings rank 5th in unintentional injury deaths.
- It is important to be trained in cardiopulmonary resuscitation (CPR) prior to performing aquatic therapy on others.
- Always check that the temperature is tolerable before applying a wrap.
- When using ice packs, place a thin cloth between the pack and the skin to prevent frostbite.
- While soaking in a tub or taking an herbal bath, reading, meditating, listening to peaceful music, or just quietly concentrating on relaxation, will help to achieve the full holistic benefits.
- It is very important to drink sufficient amounts of water to stay hydrated. The benefits of drinking water are widely recognized. Drinking pure, fresh water is essential to health.
- Caution should be taken for those with high blood pressure or cardiovascular disease. It is important to check with a physician before engaging in aquatic therapy.

Risks, Cautions, and Contraindications

It is critical to check the temperature of water prior to performing any aquatic therapy. People with impaired temperature sensation run the risk of scalding or frostbite at temperature extremes. Saunas should not be used by people with acute rheumatoid arthritis, acute infection, active tuberculosis, sexually transmitted diseases, acute mental disorders, inflammation of an inner organ or blood vessels, significant vascular changes in the brain or heart, circulatory problems, or acute cancer.

Caution should also be taken when using aquatic therapy with elderly people, and too much heat may exhaust young children (Dumas & Francesconi, 2001). The elderly should also avoid long full-body hot treatments, such as immersion baths. According to Ruoti, Morris, and Cole (1997), aquatic therapy is contraindicated in people with contagious infections, open wounds, fever, chronic ear infections, or epilepsy. Practitioners should be trained in cardiopulmonary resuscitation prior to using aquatic therapy. Patients with certain chronic illnesses should consult their physicians prior to participating in any aquatic therapy that involves changes in temperature. Caution should also be taken when using aquatic therapy on patients with the following conditions:

- Raynaud's disease
- high or low blood pressure
- diabetes mellitus
- multiple sclerosis
- pregnancy
- contagious infections.

CONCLUSION

One of the main goals of holistic health care is to promote alternative health care interventions. Aquatic therapy, or water therapy, is a unique intervention that focuses on every functional domain of an individual's life. Aquatic therapy can be performed independently, in a group setting, or one-on-one with a therapist. Many therapies have been developed to promote healing using the aquatic environment. Aquatic therapy promotes such a positive experience that many individuals continue to use it in their daily lives. One popular form of aquatic therapy is Watsu.

AQUATIC THERAPY ONLINE RESOURCES

Aquatic Resources Network
   http://www.aquaticnet.com/index.htm

Aquatic Therapy & Rehab Institute
   http://www.atri.org

Harbin Hot Springs
   http://www.harbin.org

Holistic-online.com: Hydrotherapy
   http://www.holistic-online.com/
   hydrotherapy.htm

Harbin School of Healing Arts
   http://harbinschoolofhealingarts.org

Watsu.com
   http://www.watsu.com

Worldwide Aquatic Bodywork Association
   http://www.waba.edu

EXAM QUESTIONS

CHAPTER 6
Questions 36–43

Note: Choose the one option that BEST answers each question.

36. Aquatic therapy can be used instead of pain medications for

    a. abdominal surgery.

    b. dental surgery.

    c. labor pain.

    d. children with breathing problems.

37. One well-known form of aquatic therapy is Watsu. It was developed at the Harbin Hot Springs in Northern California by Harold Dull and is based on

    a. Chinese medicine.

    b. research on different forms of aquatic therapy.

    c. Zen Shiatsu.

    d. the work of John Watson.

38. The property of water that creates a feeling of weightlessness is

    a. refraction factor.

    b. buoyancy factor.

    c. reflection factor.

    d. turbulence.

39. The method of aquatic therapy commonly used for wound healing is

    a. saunas.

    b. whirlpools.

    c. cold compresses.

    d. herbal baths.

40. Watsu aquatic therapy should be performed in

    a. hot water.

    b. cold water.

    c. tepid water.

    d. warm water.

41. A benefit seen from the use of aquatic therapy with adults with spinal cord injury is that it

    a. improves endurance.

    b. returns some level of function.

    c. reduces pain in the lower extremities.

    d. produces sensation in the muscles.

42. In the United States, among the leading causes of unintentional injury death, drowning ranks

    a. fifth.

    b. third.

    c. tenth.

    d. first.

43. Nurses should be aware that some health hazards can occur with aquatic therapy when proper safety and caution are not taken including

    a. diabetes and hypertension.

    b. hemorrhoids and rectal inflammation.

    c. legionellosis and otitis externa.

    d. back pain and multiple sclerosis.

CHAPTER 7

MUSIC THERAPY AND GUIDED IMAGERY

CHAPTER OBJECTIVE

Upon completion of this chapter, the learner will be able to describe the history and practice of music therapy and its uses as a holistic alternative and complementary therapy.

LEARNING OBJECTIVES

After studying this chapter, the learner will be able to:

1. Describe the history of music therapy.
2. Define music therapy as a holistic and complementary therapeutic modality.
3. List the principles and techniques of music therapy.
4. List the physiological and holistic benefits of music therapy as an alternative and complementary therapy.
5. Identify at least five common types of music therapy and sounds.
6. Differentiate between types of music and sounds used in music therapy.
7. Discuss the nursing responsibilities and implications associated with the use of music therapy.
8. Recognize the relationship between music therapy and guided imagery.

INTRODUCTION

Imagine for a moment songs that make you feel happy, sad, depressed, emotional, energetic, sleepy, sentimental, tense, calm, or scared. Many of us use music not just for the feelings they give us, but also for therapeutic purposes.

Music is fundamental to the body, mind, and spirit. It speaks to our inner beings and souls, and transcends time. Music therapy is a holistic modality that provides the body with energy that wakes up the inner spirit, stirs up our emotions, and promotes healing. In many cultures, music is a pure and cheap cure for many physical and emotional illnesses. For example, music therapy has been used to improve physical, mental, and restorative health and to regain speech and movement (Rankin-Box, 2001).

Music is also an art form and an expressive language for all cultures. Although music has been shown to have healing benefits, like many other natural, alternative, and complementary (NAC) therapies, science has yet to fully explain this therapeutic modality. The purpose of this chapter is to describe the practice of music therapy and relate its uses as a holistic alternative and complementary therapy. The relationship between music therapy and guided imagery will also be briefly presented.

DESCRIPTION OF MUSIC THERAPY

For generations and in every culture, music has been referred to as "medicine for the soul." However, music therapy can be defined in different ways that encompass its wide range of uses. For example, Venes, Thomas and Wilbur Taber (2013) defines "music therapy" simply as the treatment of disease, especially mental illness, with music. Keegan (2003) describes music therapy as a nonverbal communication that has been used in rituals of celebration, funerals, and ordinary transitions of daily life. She notes that music therapy involves passive relaxation combined with listening to soothing, relaxing music for the purpose of changing behavior, physiological responses, and emotions via mind modulation (Keegan, 2003).

The well-known music therapy program of the University Hospital of Cleveland (Gallagher, Huston, Nelson, Walsh, & Steele, 2001) defines music therapy as the systematic application of music in the treatment of physiological and psychosocial aspects of an illness or disability. This therapy focuses on the acquisition of nonmusical skills and behaviors, as determined by a board-certified music therapist, through systematic assessment and treatment planning. According to Burns, Harbuz, Hucklebridge, and Bunt (2001), music therapy is the use of sounds and music within an evolving relationship between client and therapist to support and encourage physical, mental, social, spiritual, and emotional well-being.

Music therapy is an established health service similar to occupational and physical therapy. Practitioners can use it to address physical, psychological, cognitive, and social functioning for clients of all ages and cultures. Health care professions are beginning to see the therapeutic values of music therapy as a powerful means of healing.

HISTORY OF MUSIC THERAPY

Music has been a part of every culture since the beginning of time. Early musical forms included chanting, praying, drumming, incantations, and mantras (Rankin-Box, 2001). The evolution of music as a therapy was based on the healing practices of many cultures.

Music therapy can be traced back to the ancient civilizations of the Egyptians, Chinese, Indians, Greeks, and Romans, as far back as 1500 B.C. (McCaffrey & Locsin, 2002; O'Kelly, 2002). Evidence of its use can be found in biblical, literary, and historical writings. O'Kelly (2002) noted that music is often described as the oldest art form to be used in healing. Apollo, a well-known Greek god, was referred to not only as the god of medicine but also as the god of music. In addition, Plato claimed that various musical "moods" or scales might successfully be prescribed for relaxation. It has also been reported that Alexander the Great's sanity was restored by music therapy (Heather, 2001).

The use of music was prominent during the Renaissance and Middle Ages. In the 1900s, many reform movements occurred, leading to the formation of the National Association for Music Therapy (NAMT) in the United States in 1950 and later, in 1958, the British Society for Music Therapy (BSMT) in the United Kingdom (UK). After the World Wars, music therapy was used in Veterans Administration Hospitals in the United States for veterans suffering from emotional and physical trauma from the wars (Karr, 1998). The recognition of the psychological, cognitive, physiological, social, and emotional benefits of music therapy by the physicians and nurses at the VA hospitals marked the true beginning of the use of music as a holistic therapy in the United States.

Today, almost all developed and some developing nations have formed their own music organizations. In the UK, for example, the Association of Professional Music Therapists (APMT) was developed in 1976 from the BSMT; this organization has played a major role in establishing state registrations of music therapists in the United States, UK, Canada, Australia, Germany, and Scandinavia. The APMT has also created a database of registered therapists, which is increasing worldwide.

Although music therapy was first introduced in the United States in the 1940s, it was not until 1998 that the American Music Therapy Association (AMTA) was formally founded as a union of the National Association for Music Therapy. According to the AMTA, music therapy is the progressive development of the therapeutic use of music in rehabilitation, special education, and community settings. By using music therapy to treat psychiatric disorders, the health care industry recognized its therapeutic possibilities. Music educators such as E. Thayer Gaston and many trained physicians played vital roles in the development of music therapy in the United States. Gaston started the first training and graduate program for music therapy in the United States (Karr, 1998). Many musicians have since composed and recorded stress-reducing musical scores that are used as alternative and supportive healing modalities.

In nursing, music started being used as a therapeutic intervention in the days of Florence Nightingale, who has been referred to as a "pioneer" of music therapy. Documentation of Nightingale's use of music therapy appears in the Florence Nightingale Museum in London and in her book *Notes on Nursing*. According to McCaffrey and Locsin (2002), Nightingale and her nurses used music therapy and musical instruments during the Crimean War to assist with the physical, social, spiritual, and emotional healing of sick and wounded soldiers. Specifically, they used voice and flute melodies for pain management and to soothe, calm, and comfort. Nightingale thought of music as an "auditory modality" that nurses could use to control the environment.

Today, nurses are increasingly recognizing, teaching, and using music therapy in practice and in the art of holistic nursing (Dossey et al., 2000; Keegan, 2003; Paterson & Zderad, 1988). Many health care professionals now use music tapes for their own relaxation as well as an adjunct for patient care.

MUSIC THERAPY PRACTICE

Principles

The therapeutic use of music is guided by six principles:

- intent
- authentic presence
- wholeness
- preference
- entrainment
- situating the client

(McCaffrey & Locsin, 2002).

These principles facilitate understanding of music therapy and its uses as a healing intervention.

Intent

The first principle, **intent**, ensures that clients are informed about the purpose of the therapy. This principle is critical because it allows the client to focus on the therapy, and it makes the second principle (authentic presence) easy to achieve. Intent gives the client an idea of what to expect during therapy and an anticipation of the possible outcomes.

An example of the principle of intent is a mother singing a lullaby to her child. The child feels the love in the mother's voice and he or she falls asleep. The intention here is loving. Intentions can also be aggressive, such as at a football match, when fans sing aggressive chants directed at an opposing team.

Authentic Presence

Authentic presence refers to a nonjudgmental acceptance of the client as a unique individual. In authentic presence, the goal is to initiate a conversation without words but with music. This allows the mind, body, and soul to use the tools from within the client to release negative energy.

Wholeness

Wholeness recognizes the idea that a person can find balance with the environment to feel complete and whole. Music is used by the client to feel as one with the environment, which is necessary for the mind-body connection.

Preference

The principle of **preference** allows the patient to select his or her own music. This is important because, in order for the client to have a positive experience with music therapy, he or she has to be willing to be in the moment. Personal selection of music allows this to occur.

Entrainment

The fifth principle, **entrainment,** explains how the body organs become engaged simultaneously or synchronically with the music. This fascinating aspect of music therapy can be illustrated by measuring a client's heart rate during music therapy. Heart rate usually slows down or speeds up to match the tone and rhythm of music. This principle, in conjunction with the client's mood and emotional state, guides the choice of music to use.

Situating the client

Situating the client is the last principle of music therapy. Prior to any use of music therapy, a proper environment should be set up. The environment should be quiet and properly lit and should contain a comfortable chair or bed for the client. A client can either sit or lie down, but he or she should be comfortable. Distractions should be removed, and the mood should be determined by the client's emotional state. The room should also be free from interruptions. An assessment is important prior to implementation of music treatment to address any complications, such as hearing difficulties.

According to O'Kelly (2002), the practice of music therapy using these principles and techniques may vary based on the choice of carefully selected or prerecorded background music, musical improvisation, songwriting by the client, receptive and recreative techniques, guided imagery, and verbal analysis of a client's imagery.

Techniques

Various techniques are used in selecting the music used to provide the therapeutic healing effect of music therapy. Examples include prerecorded background music, improvisation, songwriting, live and recorded music, and guided imagery. For example, improvisation works by providing a person with a timely vehicle for expressing emotions beyond words while affording the individual a meaningful, intimate experience of being "heard." The songwriting approach provides a medium that enhances therapeutic relationships and produces powerful means of communication (Pellitteri, 2000).

Music therapy is far more than just playing music; it is also about sound. Recorded music can be used to stimulate the senses; however, nature is also filled with sounds that can soothe, relax, and even energize a person. Sound healing can be achieved in a number of ways, including singing; speeches (both giving and listening to); karaoke; playing musical instruments; listening to bands, choirs, or orchestras; and even dancing to music and sounds. Engaging in one of the above sound activities can take our minds off our problems, help us focus our minds on other important thought processes, distract us, and ultimately relax and sedate us (Good et al., 2001). For example, loving speeches can make us relax and feel better and are extremely healing. Angry speeches have the opposite effect. Musical instruments allow us opportunities to express ourselves in unique and confident ways. They are tools that can be used to uplift our spirits and are a great way to manage stress.

One theory of how music therapy can achieve therapeutic responses claims that sensory and rhythmic stimuli that affect the limbic system through the auditory nerve and medulla evoke memories (Heather, 2001). According to Heather (2001), our bodies' atoms, molecules, cells, glands and organs all have vibrational frequencies. Sounds from outside the body stimulate sympathetic vibrations in the molecules and cells that enhance the healing process (Lewis, 2000).

Music therapy is both inspirational and therapeutic. It can conjure up memories and emotions and can serve as a source of relaxation and diversion to people who are emotionally burdened. Music can be an entertainer, a sedative, a hypnotic, an analgesic, a tranquilizer, and a spiritual counselor. Spiritually, music is used to represent different emotions, promote fellowship, prevent social isolation and, in some cultures, to march citizens to and from wars. Music can elate our spirit by giving hope and balance when nothing else is left (Harper, 2001).

Different types of music can elicit different mood responses. Certain music can help

reduce stress and feelings of isolation. Music can also contribute to the release of endorphins, the body's natural pain killers, thereby relieving pain, promoting pleasant emotions and, in turn, helping a person relax (Mazo & Parker, 2002; McCaffrey, 2000). The key is to select music to fit the individual's need and mood. Table 7-1 lists examples of types of man-made music and natural sounds.

TABLE 7-1: TYPES OF MUSIC AND SOUNDS

Types of Music (Man-Made)
- Classical
- Popular
- Country
- Rock
- Blues
- Jazz
- Instrumental: Piano, Band
- New age
- Orchestra
- Hymn
- Opera
- Folk

Types of Natural Sounds
- Rain
- Wind
- Birds
- Waves
- Wild animals
- Domestic animals
- Crickets
- Childhood sounds
- Trains

Like an orchestra, each organ, bone, and cell in the body has its own resonant frequency (Heather, 2001). Modern medicine now uses sound waves to diagnose and treat certain diseases. In fact, according to Heather (2001), scientists have suggested that listening to Mozart can improve our powers of concentration and enhance our ability to make intuitive leaps by organizing the firing patterns of neurons in the cerebral cortex. Campbell's (1997) book *The Mozart Effect* explains how different types of music can produce different responses, even to an unborn fetus. Each musical instrument, whether blended with other sounds or of its own accord can evoke a vast array of emotions, memories, and thoughts that can be very useful in boosting the immune system, reducing stress and anxiety, and promoting spiritual and physical healing.

Types of Music Therapy

Therapeutic music can be classified as sedative or stimulating. **Sedative music** can lower anxiety, pain, tension, and stress levels, resulting in decreased use of anesthetics and pain medications. **Stimulating music** can be a source of motivation, both physically and psychologically, and it can be a positive reinforcement during physical therapy and rehabilitation.

BENEFITS AND USES OF MUSIC THERAPY

The number of people who believe that music therapy can create a therapeutic and holistic healing environment for sick and stressed people is rapidly growing. Music therapy is a beneficial modality that can help people of all ages take a different approach to healing. Music therapy is used in health care settings such as hospice and palliative care, oncology units, preoperative and postoperative care units, and pediatric, obstetric, and cardiac units. It is also used in psychiatric hospitals, where it has been used to help explore personal feelings and make positive changes in mood and emotional states of the mentally ill.

Music therapy is also used in school settings. Specifically, it is used to foster the development of motor, communication, cognitive, and social abilities in children. Music therapy is particularly useful with children who have special needs. Creating, composing, singing, moving to, and listening to music can bring a wide range of cognitive, emotional, and physical abilities into focus. Music therapy can also improve social behavior, self-esteem, confidence, and communication skills in children.

Music therapy has a wide range of therapeutic benefits. According to Mazo and Parker (2002), music therapy is gaining ground as a legitimate and powerful way to treat patients with various conditions, ranging from muscle pains to different types of cancer. Marley, Searle, Chamberlain, Turnbull, and Leahy (2001), claim that music therapy has social, emotional, and psychological therapeutic benefits and can be used to stimulate creativity as well as facilitate socialization, interpersonal interactions, communication, and impulse control. Some of the physiological benefits include improved respiration, decreased blood pressure, improved cardiac output, reduced heart rate, and muscle relaxation. Music therapy is a form of sensory stimulation that provokes emotional and spiritual responses due to familiarity, predictability, and feelings of security. It also allows clients to have a sense of control, independence, and confidence. It is a medium of communication that helps refocus attention during stressful or painful procedures and long treatments or surgery. In addition, it has been used for reduction of pain and anxiety, disability, stress management, blindness, and as a diagnostic aid to identify such problems as developmental delays and expressive disorders. Specific physical uses of music therapy are to reduce the side effects of chemotherapy, reduce anxiety in patients who have experienced myocardial infarction; improve mood postoperatively in bypass patients; and assist in the management of stroke, dementia, Parkinson's disease, and anxiety, especially before or during surgery (Harper, 2001; Karr, 1998; Larkin, 2001).

The holistic value of music cannot be over-stated. Music therapy is safe, cost-effective, noninvasive, and easy to administer, so every-one can benefit from it. In fact, everyone has likely used music at some point in life to deal with an emotional, economic, spiritual, social, or political problem.

It should be noted that music therapy is not intended to be used as a cure for any of the aforementioned diseases and disorders. Rather, it can serve as a complementary or alternative therapy to aid the healing process by promoting the healing environment (Evans, 2001; Dossey et al., 2000). Table 7-2 summarizes some of the therapeutic benefits and uses of music.

TABLE 7-2: THERAPEUTIC BENEFITS AND USES OF MUSIC THERAPY

- Anxiety reduction
- Relaxation
- Pain reduction
- Sedation and hypnosis
- Decreased heart rate, blood pressure, and respiration
- Improved mood
- Improved cognitive and mental functioning
- Enhanced exercise performance
- Distraction
- Improved tolerance for procedures
- Improved satisfaction
- Stimulation of senses
- Relief of grief and sorrow

RELATED PROFESSIONAL ISSUES

For music therapy to work, the role of the certified and licensed therapist is critical. The effectiveness of music therapy depends on the relationship between the music therapist and the client. Creating a rapport is important for the healing power of music to be achieved. Patient and therapist stereotypes need to be considered prior to implementation in order to achieve the best response during treatment. The therapist needs to also have a nonjudg-mental attitude while applying the six prin-ciples of music therapy in a systematic manner (Pellitteri, 2000).

Certification and Legal and Ethical Responsibilities

Music therapists must be board certified in order to practice. According to the AMTA, the standard curriculum for becoming a music therapist includes courses in research analysis, physiology, acoustics, psychology, and music. To become a certified music therapist, one must hold a bachelor's or higher degree from one of the schools listed on the AMTA website and complete an internship at a clinical site approved by the AMTA. Once the internship is completed, the candidate is eligible to take the national certification examination that is offered by the AMTA's Certification Board of Music Therapists. Successful candidates obtain the credentials Music Therapist – Board Certified (MT-BC) (American Music Therapy Association [AMTA], n.d.).

Other types of licensures and certifications awarded in music therapy are Registered Music Therapist (RMT), Certified Music Therapist (CMT), and Advanced Certified Music Therapist (ACMT), which are based on the level of education obtained. All music thera-pists are listed on the National Music Therapy

Registry. A person who has earned a baccalaureate degree in an area other than music therapy can also become a music therapist by completing only courses required for music therapy. In such cases, the person need not earn another baccalaureate degree but can sit for the certification examination once those courses have been completed.

A certified music therapist must be reexamined every 5 years or show documentation of 100 contact hours of continuing education credits or units to continue to practice. These standards and criteria are set by the AMTA, which has official publications on the subject, including journals, monographs, bibliographies, and brochures. The AMTA has also implemented a code of ethics, standards of practice, a system of peer review, a judicial review board, and an ethics board. Every music therapist must comply with the legal and ethical standards set forth by this agency. Nurses planning to develop an independent music therapy practice must first become certified and are also required to follow the American Nurses Association and AMTA standards of practice.

Risks, Contraindications, and Client Safety Issues

Music therapy is relatively safe and has virtually no safety issues or risks associated with it. It is an effective nonpharmacological therapeutic modality that can be used by people of all ages, cultures, races, and religions. Even people with developmental delays and impairments can use and benefit from this type of therapy. However, caution should be taken with patients who have hearing difficulties. Although some claim that music therapy is contraindicated for deaf people, O'Kelly (2002) notes that these individuals, or their therapists, are able to use sign language to express their feelings and emotions. Another

safety issue can occur when music therapy is used for people who are emotionally imbalanced, such as a child who is crying or upset. Certain music may increase crying due to fear or lack of understanding. Pellitteri (2000) notes that the therapist may intervene by changing the tune of the music to change the therapeutic environment. Rankin-Box (2001) notes that music, particularly negative music, may also be contraindicated with certain health care procedures and problems. Such music should be used with caution.

According to Nightingale (1859), it is the professional responsibility of every nurse to use music therapy when appropriate to promote an environment that will enhance holistic healing. When used appropriately and safely with clients' permission, nurses can take advantage of the benefits of music therapy without any legal or ethical problems. The American Holistic Nursing Association has also noted that when music therapy is used within a holistic framework and within the scope of nursing practice, it can be used therapeutically and safely to promote self-healing, especially when used with other NAC therapies, such as relaxation and guided imagery (Dossey et al., 2000).

GUIDED IMAGERY

By combining music therapy with guided imagery, individuals can experience a variety of sensations and therapeutic benefits as they visualize peaceful scenes and images while listening to music (Cech, 2002; Dossey et al., 2000; Doherty et al., 2002; Keegan, 2003). Dossey et al. (2000) claim that music, imagery, and relaxation therapy cannot be separated. Our moods and our states of consciousness can be altered by music therapy and guided imagery. Traditionally in Eastern cultures, and now in Western cultures as well, music and guided imagery have been used to help clients focus on the seven main energy centers (chakras) believed to exist in the human body. (See Chapter 8 for a detailed description of the body's chakra points.) The use of guided imagery is a key factor in evoking and supporting transpersonal experiences (Lewis, 1998).

Guided imagery is a therapeutic modality that can be used as a tool for connecting with the unlimited capabilities of the body and mind. As a nursing intervention, it is a powerful, non-invasive, cost-effective relaxation tool that can be performed alone by a client or with guidance. It has been defined by Dossey et al. (2000) as the internal experiences of memories, dreams, fantasies, and vision, which may involve one, several, or all of the senses (visual, olfactory, tactile, gustatory, auditory, and kinesthetic), and it serves as the bridge for connecting body, mind, and spirit.

It is important to note that dreaming and daydreaming are not the same as guided imagery. Daydreaming involves fantasizing about an abstract or concrete visionary fantasy, usually spontaneously while awake, to induce inner information. In contrast, dreaming involves subconscious awareness of images, visions, and thoughts during sleep. It is a spontaneous imagery that primarily involves the visual mode, may be concrete or abstract, and provides the person with inner phenomena that can be therapeutic.

Although guided imagery has been in existence since the beginning of shamanic cultures and civilization, one of the most innovative works on the subject was developed in the last century by Helen Bonny, a music-centered psychotherapist. In the 1970s, Bonny and her colleague Louise Savary used guided imagery and music to develop the physiological and psychological aspect of guided imagery

and music therapy uses in many health care situations today (Bernatzky, 2003; Cech, 2002; Doherty et al., 2002; Elliott, 2003; Keegan, 2003; Laurion, 2003; Wall, 2002).

As far back as 1973, Bonny and Savary addressed the relationship between music therapy and guided imagery in their book *Music and Your Mind*. Bonny and Savary later founded the Institute for Music and Imagery, an educational and research institute dedicated to furthering the use of music and the art of imagery as agents of healing (Bonny, 1983; Doherty et al., 2002; Dossey et al., 2000). Bonny's innovative approach to listening to music combined with the use of imagery was called guided imagery and music (GIM). GIM is the conscious use of imagery and music to evoke relaxation. It allows for self-healing through self-exploration, self-understanding, growth, and transformation. In GIM, a person's imagination can come to conscious awareness while he or she listens to music in a relaxed state with or without a guide. With the presence of a guide, the experience can be integrated into real life.

Music therapy and guided imagery are both anxiety-reducing techniques that can be used in various health care settings, including pre-operative and postoperative care units and labor and delivery units. Specifically, Keegan (2003) describes how guided imagery can be combined with other complementary therapies and used daily by staff in acute and critical care hospital environments to help decrease anxiety. In addition to GIM, several cd's have been developed that use voice-guided imagery to help the listener evoke the relaxation response. The cd's help the client to learn the skills of relaxation and apply these skills to stressful events, such as surgery or preterm labor (Elliott, 2003; Laurion, 2003; Schiedermayer, 2000).

CONCLUSION

Music therapy is fundamental to our body, mind, and spirit. For generations and in every culture, music has been referred to as "medicine for the soul." The therapeutic use of music however is guided by six principles: intent, authentic presence, wholeness, preference, entrainment, and situation of the client.

Music therapy is both inspirational and therapeutic. It can be used as an entertainer, a tranquilizer, a sedative, a hypnotic, an analgesic, and as a spiritual and emotional counselor. One theory of how music therapy (different sounds) can achieve therapeutic responses is the effect of the sensory and rhythmic stimuli on the limbic system through the auditory nerve and medulla. Music therapy is often used with guided imagery which is another therapeutic modality which uses memories, dreams, fantasies, and vision in its healing process. Although the practice of music therapy and guided imagery are safe and cost-effective, they are not intended to be used as a cure but as a complementary and alternative therapy to aid the healing process.

MUSIC THERAPY ONLINE RESOURCES

American Music Therapy Association
http://www.musictherapy.org

Institute for Music and Neurologic Function
http://musictherapy.imnf.org

Music Therapy at the University Hospitals of Cleveland
http://www.musicasmedicine.com

World Federation of Music Therapy
http://www.musictherapyworld.net

EXAM QUESTIONS

CHAPTER 7
Questions 44–52

Note: Choose the one option that BEST answers each question.

44. The first nurse to use and teach the use of music therapy in nursing is

    a. Jean Watson.
    b. Rosemary Parse.
    c. Florence Nightingale.
    d. Dorothy Orem.

45. For the purpose of healing, music therapy is guided by six principles. One principle is

    a. authentic presence.
    b. expect presence.
    c. anticipation presence.
    d. nonjudgmental presence.

46. As a principle of music therapy, entrainment is defined as

    a. the process by which a person can find balance with the environment to feel complete and whole.
    b. the process by which the body organs become engaged simultaneously or synchronically with music.
    c. recognition that a person is one with the sound and tone of music.
    d. a positive experience with music therapy and the willingness to be in the moment.

47. An example of a natural sound is

    a. popular music.
    b. blues music.
    c. relaxing sound.
    d. wave sound.

48. Music is a holistic therapy that provides us with energy that awakens our inner spirits and stirs up our emotions. Music therapy can be considered

    a. a yin-yang phenomenon.
    b. a dreaming and daydreaming experience.
    c. an inspirational and therapeutic experience.
    d. a memories experience.

49. Therapeutic benefits of music therapy include

    a. treatment of gastrointestinal problems.
    b. blood pressure reduction.
    c. treatment of infection.
    d. treatment of memory loss.

50. All certified music therapists hold

    a. diplomas.
    b. bachelor's degrees.
    c. master's degrees.
    d. doctoral degrees.

51. The NAC therapy that is most closely linked with music therapy is

    a. meditation.
    b. reflexology.
    c. therapeutic touch.
    d. guided imagery.

77

continued on next page

52. The psychotherapist who developed GIM, the innovative combination of music therapy and guided imagery, is

   a. Louise Savary.

   b. Florence Nightingale.

   c. Helen Bonny.

   d. James Goodman.

CHAPTER 8

YOGA AND MEDITATION

CHAPTER OBJECTIVE

Upon completion of this chapter, the learner will be able to discuss the history and practice of yoga and meditation therapy and their uses as holistic alternative and complementary therapies.

LEARNING OBJECTIVES

After studying this chapter, the learner will be able to:

1. Describe the history of yoga.
2. Identify at least five different types of yoga.
3. List the principles and techniques of yoga.
4. Define yoga, hypnosis, and meditation as holistic alternative and complementary therapeutic modalities.
5. List the physiological and holistic benefits of meditation as a natural alternative and complementary (NAC) therapy.
6. List the physiological and holistic benefits of yoga as a NAC therapy.
7. Discuss the nursing responsibilities and implications associated with the use of yoga and meditation.
8. Indicate the meanings of ten Sanskrit words commonly used in yoga.

INTRODUCTION

Yoga is not an organized religion; however, it can be used to improve one's relationship with oneself and with one's spiritual being. The spiritual aspect of yoga is strictly based on an individual (Steinberg, 2002). It is also an art, a science, a philosophy, and a lifestyle (Payne, 1997). Yoga is a psychophysio-logical discipline with roots that date back 5,000 years or more. Founded by Patanjali, the practice of yoga includes standing, sitting, balancing, and breathing poses, as well as twists and inversion movements, each designed to offer particular health and spiritual benefits. It is a unique way of life and a holistic practice that incorporates meditation, exercises, breathing, and spirituality to achieve the goal of harmony and balance. It is also a form of exercise that allows the body to use breathing to connect the body and the mind. Yoga is fast becoming popular (Saper, Eisenberg, Davis, Culpepper, & Phillips, 2004).

Meditation is the art of focusing attention so completely on one thing that a person no longer focuses on everything else around him or her. It has a religious and philosophical background. Although meditation can be practiced alone, it is frequently used with relaxation exercises, yoga, and other types of alternative therapies. Like yoga, meditation is a very effective method of relaxation. But unlike hypnosis, which is a passive experience, meditation is an active process directed toward balancing the mind, body, and spirit.

When yoga is practiced with meditation, there is a profound spiritual benefit that can transcend the ordinary physical and mental benefits. The purpose of this chapter is to discuss the practices of yoga and meditation and relate their uses as holistic alternative and complementary therapies. Although meditation and hypnotherapy are discussed in terms of their relationship to yoga, this chapter focuses on yoga.

HISTORY AND CHARACTERISTICS OF YOGA

Although the exact origin of yoga is unknown, yoga practice has been recorded in Asia, specifically in India. Patanjali, who is referred to as the "Founder of Yoga," compiled the earliest known text on yoga and set down the well-known theories and practice of yoga called Yoga Sutra. The book *Yoga Sutra,* originally written in Sanskrit, contains about 196 aphorisms, which have been developed into what are now called the eight steps of classical yoga. Through misconceptions, yoga was believed to be rooted in the religion of Hinduism. Today, however, it is now known that Hinduism's structure evolved much later than yoga and it incorporated some of the practices of yoga as well as those of other Eastern religions and cultures (Schaeffer, 1999; American Yoga Association, 2005a).

Yoga was introduced in the United States in the late 1800s. However, it was not until the 1960s, after yoga was introduced in the media, that it began to be recognized by the public. It was American youths who first began to experiment with yoga as mind-body flexibility and twisting workout exercises. Although many people still erroneously view yoga as merely another form of exercise, yoga has gained acceptance and respect as a valuable method for helping manage stress and improve health and well-being. In the last 40 years, Americans have begun to implement yoga in mainstream health care in a number of ways, including research initiatives by the National Center for Complementary and Alternative Medicine and the American Yoga Association.

DESCRIPTION

Yoga is a system of physical and mental exercises that include breathing techniques, meditation, and postures. It was born of a desire to achieve greater personal freedom, holistic health, longer life, and heightened self-understanding. According to Colin (1997), the word "yoga" comes from the ancient Sanskrit root word *yug,* which means "to unify or join together." Yoga, therefore, means to bind, join, attach, and direct one's attention to union or communion with some higher being.

The practice of yoga includes standing, sitting, balancing, and breathing poses, called *asanas,* as well as twists and inversion movements, each designed to offer particular health and spiritual benefits (Garfinkel & Schumacher, 2000; Malhotra et al., 2002; Ram, Holloway, & Jones, 2003). Through these asanas and exercises, yoga creates body, mind, and spirit harmony and promotes relaxation. It is a unique holistic practice and way of life (Payne, 1997).

The exercises used in yoga are designed to ease muscle tension, tone internal organs, and improve the flexibility of the body's joints and ligaments (mobility). Each posture in yoga is performed slowly. Violent movements are discouraged in yoga because they can cause the buildup of lactic acid and fatigue. The key to performing yoga is to learn the art of proper breathing, which includes breathing in through the nose and concentrating on exhalation rather than inhalation to cleanse the lungs of stale air. This art of proper breathing assists with the elimination of toxins from the body. Complete harmony through yoga also requires proper relaxation and diet. Meditation, which is a state of consciousness, is an important technique that is used in all types of yoga. Proper thinking and meditation help to calm the mind and focus mental energy inward. Meditation also helps to relieve stress and replenish energy.

The first step in appreciating and learning yoga is to be willing to appreciate the language and context in which yoga is presented. Yoga contains approximately 196 axioms, maxims, or aphorisms built around the ancient Indian language of Sanskrit (see Table 8-1).

According to the American Yoga Association (2005a) in his book *Yoga Sutras*, Patanjali includes some of the principles of what is called today "classical yoga," which includes the types and paths of classical yoga. The seven "Principles of Man" are

1. the lower body, which is the physical body
2. the astral body, which is the outside aura that surrounds the physical body
3. the prana, or vital force, which represents universal energy
4. the instinctive mind, which deals with how we think about bad things, such as committing a sin
5. the intellectual mind, which represents the ability to think intelligently
6. the spiritual mind, which is the godlike unconscious good characteristics
7. level of optimal achievement, which is the highest level that one has to achieve to acquire complete spiritual godliness or wholeness

(Astin, Shapiro, Eisenberg, & Forys, 2003).

These seven principles help to explain the philosophy of this holistic practice.

Eight Steps of Classical Yoga

In addition to the "Principles of Man," Patanjali discussed eight limbs, or steps, of yoga. The eight steps of classical yoga are listed here.

1. *Yama* means restraint from violence, lying, stealing, casual sex, and harsh words, thoughts, and deeds in life.

2. *Niyama* means observance of purity, contentment, tolerance, and remembrance.
3. *Asana* deals with physical exercise or postures.
4. *Pranayama* relates to the preparation for meditation. It regulates life forces through channeling of breathing techniques.
5. *Pratyahara* deals with meditation, or the withdrawal of the mind from the domination of the senses.
6. *Dharana* deals with concentration, or being able to hold the mind on one object for a specified time.
7. *Dhyana* is meditation attention focused internally and externally at the same time.
8. *Samadhi* deals with absorption or realization of the essential nature of self. It is a state in which the practitioner is one with the object of meditation.

Yama and Niyama are sometimes referred to as the do's and don'ts of yoga, whereas Dharana, Dhyana, and Samadhi are stages of a continual process.

Types and Paths of Yoga

Many different types of yoga are practiced today; they may be used alone or together. For example, in Hinduism, a combination of steps and types of yoga are used to achieve harmony and closeness to a higher being (Schaeffer, 1998; Steinberg, 2002). Some types include Hatha, Raja, Jnana, Bhakti, Karma, Mantra, Tantra, and Laya. However, classical yoga generally follows four paths.

- Jnana represents the yoga of knowledge and wisdom.
- Bhakti is the yoga of selfless love and the path of devotion to the divine.
- Karma is the path of yoga in action.
- Raja represents the final path of self-control.

Jnana yoga suggests that, through meditation, the mind withdraws along with emotions from perceiving life in a deluded way.

TABLE 8-1: COMMON SANSKRIT WORDS USED IN YOGA

- **Agni:** fire; the god of fire
- **Agni kriya:** an advanced breathing exercise involving manipulation of the diaphragm while the breath is held out
- **Agnya (Ajna) chakra:** state of consciousness in which intuitive wisdom resides; represented in the body by the spot between the eyebrows
- **Anahat chakra:** energy center in the subtle body associated with the heart
- **Asan, Asana:** a position, posture, or movement in yoga exercise
- **Buddhidhyana:** intellectual meditation
- **Chakras:** centers of energy that are connected with the physical body at various locations along the spinal column
- **Dharana:** concentration; the sixth of the eight stages of classical yoga
- **Dharma:** work, duty, or destiny
- **Dhyana:** meditation or contemplation; the seventh of the eight stages of classical yoga
- **Guru:** spiritual teacher
- **Hinduism:** one of the major religions of India
- **Humming breath:** a breathing exercise that involves a short inhalation and long exhalation while making a humming sound
- **Kashmir Shaivism:** a school of yoga philosophy that recognizes the essential unity of everything in the universe
- **Mantra, Mantram:** a sound formula of particular syllables repeated by yogis to produce a change in consciousness
- **Namaste, Namaskar:** Indian greeting (latter is more respectful)
- **Om, Aum:** the sound from which all other sounds come; a mantram often used before meditation
- **Patanjali:** Sanskrit grammarian who compiled and systematized all ancient techniques and theories of Yoga into aphorisms called *Yoga Sutras*; this system is generally known as classical yoga
- **Pranayama:** breathing techniques
- **Prasad:** food or other offerings to higher being as part of a devotional service that are distributed to the participants afterward
- **Pratyahara:** withdrawal of the mind from the senses; an essential first step in meditation and the fifth of the eight stages of classical yoga
- **Primiti:** supersubjective consciousness
- **Rajas:** one of the three qualities of nature (gunas), which manifest as activity, restlessness, and passion
- **Sahasrara:** Chakra located just above the top of the head
- **Vigu:** energy
- **Yamas:** literally, "restraints:" nonviolence, truthfulness, non stealing, celibacy
- **Yoga Sutras:** a collection of concise aphorisms for the practice of yoga as collected and set down by Patanjali

(American Yoga Association, 2005d)

Bhakti yoga centers on emotional fulfillment. People who practice this yoga form pour out their hearts' love and adoration and share their deepest thoughts and concerns with the higher being until a continual flow of awareness moves between devotion and the Lord.

Karma yoga includes conscious focus on the spiritual and away from the ego and self. It is a part of nature and promotes zen-like tranquility. This type of yoga involves dedication to a selfless, altruistic service to humanity, and is said to be the most authentic way to progress in the spiritual life.

Raja means royal. Raja yoga involves the use of meditation to direct one's life force in order to bring the mind and emotion into self-control and balance.

Most elements of modern yoga are derived from **Hatha yoga.** The word "hatha" is derived from the word *Ha,* meaning sun, and *tha,* meaning moon. This type of yoga focuses the body's inner feelings until they are perfectly balanced by dealing with opposite emotions. Hatha yoga includes using controlled breathing, prescribed postures (asanas), and meditation to enhance prana (the life force).

According to Steinberg (2002), **iyengar yoga** is a type of Hatha yoga that is commonly practiced in the United States. Deeply grounded in the ancient yoga tradition, iyengar yoga emphasizes standing poses for strength, alignment, concentration, and stability and the use of props to facilitate learning how to use yoga to manage stress and certain illnesses.

Mantra yoga involves meditation and chanting of words or phrases, and **tantra** yoga focuses on dynamic aspects of divinity called *shakti,* or the "cosmic mother" (Mystic World Fellowship, 1999; Riley, 2004).

YOGA PRACTICE

Yoga is based on three main concepts or components: meditation, exercise, and breathing. The art of connecting the practice and techniques of certain exercises, breathing, and meditation makes yoga a unique holistic alternative and complementary therapeutic modality. The three techniques are structured to facilitate the glandular systems of the body, as a result, bringing the body and mind into harmony and balance. Breathing is the most important aspect of the practice. The breathing technique is theoretically considered the source of life in the body. Breathing exercises and postures prepare the mind for the meditation that ultimately enables achievement of peace and wholeness (Mystic World Fellowship, 1999; Schaeffer, 1999).

Breathing

The key to yoga is learning the art of proper breathing, which includes breathing in through the nose and concentrating on exhalation rather than inhalation to cleanse the lungs of stale air. Yoga breathing begins with a technique commonly referred to as "belly breath," which is an introductory exercise that teaches diaphragmatic breathing by emphasizing movement of the lower abdomen. Complete breathing, used during yoga, involves exercises of even inhalation and exhalation using all respiratory muscles. Proper breathing assists with elimination of toxins in the body (Holistic-online.com, n.d.-e).

Poses

The breathing exercises of yoga are used in conjunction with the asanas, or poses. The name of each pose ends with the term "asana." Some of the postures of yoga include prayer, standing, forward, backward, pushups, lunge, lying down, headstand, shoulder stand, inversions, seated, twisted, and balancing.

Warm Up

Before starting any yoga exercise, a person should perform warm-up exercises. A 12-part warm-up exercise called the *sun salutation* is often recommended (Colin, 1997). This warm-up instills a feeling of balance and harmony by moving the vertebrae into different postures, including the prayer pose, arch back, bend over, leg back, push up, lower chest to the floor, chest arch, inverted V, lunge forward, forehead to knees, stretch back, and return to start.

Meditation

Meditation is the art of focusing attention so completely on one thing that a person no longer focuses on everything else around him or her. Although it can be used alone, meditation is frequently used with relaxation exercises, yoga, and other types of natural, alternative, and complementary (NAC) therapies. Through meditation, one can learn to control his or her body. The experience is similar to the one a person has in a movie theater, where attention is focused on the movie for an extended amount of time, and other stimuli are blocked out.

One of the steps of classical yoga is dhyana, which means meditation. According to Steinberg (2002), dhyana meditation is not simply sitting, closing the eyes, and emptying the mind, but it is a cosmic consciousness of harmony of the body and mind. Before getting to the step of dhyana in classical Hatha or iyengar yoga, asana and pranayama must be achieved.

Meditation can be beneficial to everyone, especially people with very stressful lifestyles. It is a very effective method of relaxation that calms the overactive mind and improves concentration and the ability to tap into one's inner self.

Meditation can be practiced at any time of day and anywhere, inside or outside. To practice meditation alone, one simply requires a warm space free from noise, distraction, and clutter. An environment of natural beauty, such as by the ocean or on top of a hill, is particularly beneficial for meditation. Any place that can provide a peaceful state of mind is feasible. A comfortable sitting position, such as the cross-legged position, is also highly recommended for meditation. Like yoga, the key to meditation is breathing. Techniques for achieving a state of meditation faster include staring into a flame for about one minute while trying not to blink and repeating a mantra or rhythm. Focusing on the mental and spiritual energy from the body chakras helps keep the process grounded.

The use of chakras is not unique to the practices of yoga and meditation. Chakras originated from many Eastern health care practices and philosophies. Chakras are defined as the seven energy centers in our bodies and are the basis of holistic healing therapies, such as yoga and meditation. Chakras are the openings through which life energy flows into and out of the aura. The functions of these centers are to vitalize the physical body and to bring about self-consciousness. According to the American Institute of Holistic Theology, the seven chakras are bioenergetic activity radiating from bundles of energy clusters, or vortices, that start at the base of the spine and continue upward to the crown of the head. Although chakra energies can be perceived with specific assessment tools, they contain no substantive mass or substance of their own.

It should be noted that meditation is not always easy to achieve. However, simple meditation can be accomplished by sitting in a comfortable position, either in a chair or on the floor, with the back and head straight. Warming up with a couple of deep breaths and closing the eyes can be beneficial. In breathing, it is recommended to inhale through the nose and exhale through the mouth. Focus on the breath as "cool air in" and "warm air out." If the mind wanders during this process, gently refocus the breathing by counting breaths. For example, count up to four and then repeat, over and over again. Count only during inhalation while focusing on one object.

Chakras are the key to achieving the full benefit of holistic alternative and complementary therapies, such as yoga and meditation. The first chakra, which resides in the tailbone or sacrum, called the Muladhara, is the center of innocence and sexuality. Chakra number two, Svadisthana, is the chakra of creativity. The third chakra is called Manipura (Nubhi), the peace chakra. The fourth chakra, Anahata, is the chakra of the heart, love, and compassion. The fifth chakra, Visuddha, is the chakra of collectivity and diplomacy. The sixth chakra, which is the chakra of forgiveness, is called Agnya (Ajna). The last chakra, Sahasrara, is the chakra of integration and it is housed on top of the head.

Hypnosis

Unlike yoga and meditation, hypnosis is a condition or state of being put to sleep. The primary purpose of hypnosis is to induce sleep. The process is characterized by a marked susceptibility to suggestion and considerable loss of willpower and sensation. Achieved through hypnotherapy, hypnosis can be used by a trained hypnotist for the treatment of mental and physical diseases or conditions. Hypnotics are drugs or other agents that are used to produce sleep, such as benzodiazepines or barbiturates. Hypnosis can only be practiced and administered by a trained hypnotist or hypnotherapist. Unlike hypnosis, which is a passive experience, meditation and yoga are active processes directed toward balancing the mind, body, and spirit.

Benefits of Yoga

All aspects of one's life – work, play, relationships, ego, mind, decisions, health, habits – can benefit from a dedicated practice of

yoga (Steinberg, 2002). Yoga is beneficial in controlling breathing; stretching and strengthening muscles; improving posture; inducing relaxation; improving sleep, digestion, and concentration; and focusing the mind (Schaeffer, 2002b). Some other benefits of yoga include stress reduction, increased flexibility and self-awareness, decreased blood pressure, muscle relaxation, clear thinking, reduced irritability, and relief from stress headaches. When yoga is practiced with meditation, there is a profound spiritual benefit that can transcend the ordinary physical and mental benefits (Bright, 2002). The mystical benefits of yoga and meditation place an individual in touch with his or her intuition, creativity, and other aspects of self of which he or she might not previously have been aware.

The yoga philosophy of health and wellness considers that most diseases are due to insufficient life forces (prana or energy), either in the body as a whole or a blockage to one part of the body. This deficiency often leads to lowered body resistance or immunity to disease. The therapeutic purpose of yoga is to restore or maintain physical health and the life force or energy. The real power of yoga, however, lies in its strength as a holistic method of psychospiritual healing, leading to inner peace, clarity and, ultimately, enlightenment and freedom. Yoga helps bring balance and harmony to the mind, body, and spirit. It is also helpful in calming, nurturing, and managing fatigue and low energy.

Since yoga was introduced to the Western world, it has been used as a holistic and complementary therapy for many conditions. Yoga has been proven to increase cardiac efficiency, slow respiration rate, improve fitness, promote relaxation, and reduce stress and anxiety. As a complementary therapy, yoga has been used to manage the effects of such conditions as cancer, acne, chronic fatigue syndrome, depression, fibromyalgia, heart disease, infertility, menopause, headaches, anemia, angina, diabetes, arthritis, asthma, migraines, acquired immunodeficiency syndrome, addictions, smoking, and stress. Garfinkel et al. (1998) report on the effectiveness of yoga in the management of pain, joint, and bone diseases and stress-related illnesses (Jacobs et al., 2004; Kleiner, 2002; Labarthe & Ayala, 2002; Manocha, 2003; McIver, O'Halloran, & McGartland, 2004). However, yoga is not a cure for any of the aforementioned conditions. In addition, it is recommended that one should avoid smoking, alcohol, and caffeine and follow certain recommended diets daily to get the proper benefits of yoga (American Yoga Association, 2005a).

RELATED PROFESSIONAL ISSUES

Education, Certification, and Licensure

Although there are many yoga retreats in the United States, there are no national programs for teaching yoga. However, schools exist internationally, mostly in the Eastern cultures (for example, in Kashmir, India). For many years, the tradition of yoga was simply transmitted from teachers to students or passed on from generation to generation. Today, however, yoga skills can be acquired in other ways, such as by training with a yoga master, teacher, or instructor or attending a yoga school.

Because no national programs exist, there are also no national certification processes. Currently, there are also no set educational requirements or standards for certification or licensure as a yoga instructor. Many people learn to teach yoga the traditional way – from their teachers or masters. However, a number of individual schools across the country certify their graduates, according to their own standards and requirements. Furthermore, health

and exercise facilities and schools expect their yoga instructors to follow certain standards and requirements to be able to practice.

Although anyone can practice yoga, the American Yoga Association (2005b) recommends that a yoga instructor maintain certain ethical standards and have specified amounts of daily regular practice in some of the following areas

- yoga exercise
- breathing techniques
- meditation
- regular contact with a teacher
- study of important yoga text
- ethical behavior
- understanding or practice (not a mandate) of a healthy vegetarian diet
- training on basic anatomy and the effects of yoga techniques
- ability to separate yoga from religion.

Legal and Ethical Responsibilities

Yoga is a unique alternative and complementary therapy that should not be taught without years of training and dedication to the practice. Yoga involves a serious everyday commitment not only to oneself but to the practice. An ethical yoga teacher conducts classes in a responsible and safe environment without pushing students beyond their limits. Legally and ethically, anyone taking the responsibility to teach others how to use yoga and meditation should be able to vary the techniques according to the students' abilities (Payne, 1997).

According to Payne (1997) and the American Yoga Association (2005b), ethical behavior expected of actual or potential yoga masters, teachers, instructors, or students should include taking responsibility for knowing and practicing the five yamas (the first step in classical yoga) and the five niyamas (the second step of classical yoga). These two steps are among the eight steps of classical yoga written by Patanjali thousands of years ago. The remaining six steps – asana, pranayama, pratyahara, dharana, dhyana, and samadhi – cannot be achieved without the first two ethical principles. The meanings of these steps were discussed earlier in this chapter and can be located in Table 8-1, which presents some key Sanskrit terms. Although a very close relationship is often formed between yoga mentors and their students, sexual involvement with students is absolutely prohibited in the practice of yoga (Christensen, 2003).

Ethical and legal responsibilities for nurses vary by state. Nurses who are considering incorporating yoga into their practice should check with the board of nursing in their state and with the American Yoga Association before doing so. In addition, they should undergo proper training and follow the ethical guidelines of classical yoga as set down by Patanjali.

Cautions, Contraindications, and Client Safety Issues

According to the American Yoga Association (2005c), people with a history of back injury, surgery, disk problems, severe arthritis, or uncontrolled hypertension should not practice yoga without first consulting their physicians. It is recommended that beginners only practice yoga under the supervision of a trained and certified yoga teacher or instructor. This is essential if one suffers from a chronic condition, such as those listed above. Yoga should not be performed by anyone suffering from a medical condition that involves mobility. To get the proper benefits of yoga, one should avoid smoking, alcohol, and caffeine.

When attempting any yoga exercises or asanas, it is important not to force any posture. It is also important for teachers to vary the techniques according to each student's ability and to be able to advise students appropriately.

Patients with certain conditions, such as hypertension, arthritis, or back problems, should get medical clearance prior to performing yoga. Caution should also be used if a student has a history of detached retina, glaucoma, heart disease, or stroke. Certain poses are contraindicated in patients with these medical issues (American Yoga Association, 2005c).

Finally, according to Schaeffer (2002f) and Christensen (2003), some yoga exercises are not recommended for women who are pregnant or nursing, children under 16 years of age, people with hernia or disk problems, and elderly people with chronic or recurring conditions. These students should be referred to their physicians for advice before beginning a program. Schaeffer (2002f) notes that gentle yoga can be used to alleviate the minor discomforts of pregnancy but only if properly supervised. In such cases, certain poses should be avoided. For more information about caution and safety issues associated with yoga, visit the American Yoga Association web site.

CONCLUSION

Yoga and meditation, in some cultures and religions, are a unique way of life. Yoga is not an organized religion but a holistic practice that incorporates meditation, exercises, breathing, and spirituality to achieve harmony and balance. Meditation, on the other hand, is the art of focusing attention so completely on one thing that we can no longer focus on anything else around us. Although meditation can be used alone, it is frequently used with relaxation exercises as they are both very effective methods of relaxation.

Yoga practice includes standing, sitting, balancing, and breathing poses called asanas. There are different types and paths of yoga which require strict dedication from the practitioner. All yoga practices goes through certain steps and techniques that involve the use of the energy channels, the body's chakras, and the use of meditation.

YOGA WEB RESOURCES

American Yoga Association
   http://www.americanyogaassociation.org

Anusara Yoga
   http://www.anusara.com

A World of Yoga
   http://www.yogaworld.org

Introduction to Yoga
   http://www.introductiontoyoga.com

Satyananda Yoga
   http://www.satyananda.net

The Seven Bodies
   http://www.home.att.net/~meditation/seven.
   html

Yoga Directory
   http://www.yogadirectory.com

Yoga Forums
   http://www.yogaforums.com

Yoga as a Complementary Health Approach
   http://nccam.nih.gov/news/multimedia/
   infographics/yoga

EXAM QUESTIONS

CHAPTER 8
Questions 53–61

Note: Choose the one option that BEST answers each question.

53. The founder of yoga is

    a. Parse.

    b. Christensen.

    c. St. John.

    d. Patanjali.

54. Unlike hypnosis, meditation and yoga are considered

    a. passive processes.

    b. active processes.

    c. passive processes with the use of an agent.

    d. active processes with the use of an agent.

55. In the United States, yoga was primarily recognized by the public after the media introduced the practice in the

    a. 1800s.

    b. 1900s.

    c. 1960s.

    d. 1990s.

56. Yoga generally follows four paths. Which of the following terms is not one of the four paths of yoga?

    a. Jnana

    b. Hatha

    c. Karma

    d. Raja

57. The therapeutic purpose of yoga is to restore or maintain physical and mental health as well as

    a. restore broken bones.

    b. restore the prana life force or energy.

    c. prevent smoking.

    d. prevent unethical behaviors.

58. A type of yoga that is commonly practiced in the United States and is deeply grounded in the ancient yoga tradition is called

    a. manta yoga.

    b. iyengar yoga.

    c. bhaki yoga.

    d. karma yoga.

59. Which of the following practices is not a part of yoga?

    a. Asana

    b. Meditation

    c. Hypnosis

    d. Breathing

60. A competent yoga teacher or student must have a certain amount of daily practice in the yoga philosophy, including

    a. practicing yoga as a religion.

    b. eating a vegetarian diet for life.

    c. showing ethical behaviors.

    d. practicing hypnotherapy.

continued on next page

61. A Sanskrit word used in yoga that represents the most respectful greeting is

   a. pranayama.

   b. sahasrara.

   c. Yoga Sutras.

   d. namaskar.

CHAPTER 9

TOUCH THERAPY: MASSAGE AND THERAPEUTIC TOUCH

CHAPTER OBJECTIVE

Upon completion of this chapter, the learner will be able to describe the history and practice of touch therapies, such as massage therapy and Therapeutic Touch, their uses as holistic alternative and complementary therapies.

LEARNING OBJECTIVES

After studying this chapter, the learner will be able to:

1. Describe the history of touch therapy.
2. Describe massage therapy as a holistic complementary therapeutic modality.
3. List the physiological and holistic benefits of massage therapy as an alternative and complementary therapy.
4. List the types and techniques of massage therapy.
5. Identify at least five common types of massage therapy.
6. Explain Therapeutic Touch as a holistic complementary therapeutic modality.
7. Identify the physiological and holistic benefits of Therapeutic Touch as an alternative and complementary therapy.
8. List the four steps of Therapeutic Touch.
9. Differentiate between the various types of touch therapy.
10. Discuss the nursing responsibilities and implications associated with massage and Therapeutic Touch.

INTRODUCTION

The recent drive for the use of various natural, alternative, and complementary (NAC) therapies in health care today has resulted in the revisitation of many of the various therapeutic modalities originally practiced by shamans and cultural leaders since the beginning of civilization. In addition, as health care continues to be an expanding yet expensive business, patients are searching for less costly and less invasive procedures to manage diseases. NAC therapies are among the options (Huebscher & Shuler, 2003) and are now becoming more and more popular not only for treatment of diseases but for prevention of stress-producing illnesses. One such practice is touch therapy. Some other types of touch therapy not discussed in this chapter are chiropractic, Jin shin, and Reiki.

Touch therapy is a unique therapy because the same touch can have different meanings to different cultures. The concept of touch is also dynamic. Some cultures may value and embrace physical contact, such as with massage therapy, whereas others may value the nonphysical contact of Therapeutic Touch (Krieger, 1999; Spence & Olson, 1997).

The purpose of this chapter is to discuss the practice of touch therapy and relate its uses as a holistic alternative and complementary therapy. Two forms of touch therapy, massage therapy and Therapeutic Touch, will be discussed in detail.

HISTORY OF TOUCH THERAPY

One of the oldest therapies known to man, both in the secular and religious worlds, is the act of touch. Documentation of its use can be found in a number of literary, medical, and historic sources and in the bible. Touch therapies, such as Healing Touch, caring touch, Kangaroo Care, massage therapy, Therapeutic Touch, shiatzu, and reflexology, have been used by all cultures. Because not all individuals or cultures embrace the concept of physical contact with touch, some use touch indirectly. For example, in Therapeutic Touch, the modern form of the ancient practice of "laying on of the hands," practitioners use touch indirectly. Although Therapeutic Touch is a relatively new therapeutic modality, touch therapy is as old as civilization itself.

Evidence of touch therapy can be found in the history of every culture since the beginning of civilization. Like many other NAC therapies, the origin of touch therapy can be traced back to the Egyptians, Chinese, Indians, Polynesians, Native Americans, Greeks, Romans, and Africans. It was used in early shaman practices, in traditional healing practices, and in the practices of almost all religions, including Christianity. The uses of touch therapies as healing arts has been documented by Cohen (1998); Dossey et al. (2000); Huebscher and Shuler (2003); Molloy (2000); Spence and Olson (1997); and others.

Nurses have used touch therapy since the beginning of nursing practice and the days of Florence Nightingale. Today, many unique types of touch therapeutics exist, such as Kangaroo Care, which is specifically used to decrease high mortality rates among premature infants by providing skin-to-skin contact in the form of healing touch, back rubs, hugs, and caring touch. Caring touch is another type of touch therapy that is done by nurses with an intention (motivation) that involves empathy and concern. Despite the many variations of touch therapy in different cultures, the basic principles remain the same: to stimulate or change the energy channel of the body and help to restore or maintain balance.

DESCRIPTION AND TYPES OF TOUCH THERAPY

The term *touch therapy* refers to a broad range of techniques used by practitioners that involve putting the hands on or near the body to assist a client toward optimal functioning or healing (Molloy, 2000). Some types of touch therapies are massage therapy (therapeutic massage), Therapeutic Touch, shiatzu, and reflexology (see Chapter 5). As previously discussed (see Chapter 6), shiatzu is a form of touch therapy in which the practitioner uses the thumb or heel of the hand to apply deep pressure along the energy lines, or chakras.

Healing Touch is another form of touch therapy that was developed by a nurse named Janet Mentgen. The practice is defined by Healing Touch International (1998) as a relaxing, nurturing energy therapy. Healing Touch providers use gentle, noninvasive touch to influence and support the energy system within and around the body. The goal of Healing Touch is to restore harmony and balance within the human energy system or field. This goal supports the client's self-healing process of becoming whole in body, mind, emotion, and spirit. Healing Touch is a biofield therapy that is approved and endorsed by the American Holistic Nurses Association.

Massage therapy, or therapeutic massage, is the process of using one's hands to directly apply pressure and motion to the skin and underlying muscle of a client for the purposes of physical and psychological relaxation, improvement of circulation, relief of sore muscles, and other therapeutic purposes. This commonly used form of touch therapy will be described in detail later in this chapter.

In 1972, Dolores Krieger developed a touch therapy called Therapeutic Touch. In this practice, a practitioner moves his or her hands through a client's energy fields for the purpose of assessment and treatment of energy field imbalance. The practitioner does not actually touch the client in this therapy. Therapeutic Touch is not as widely used as some other forms of touch therapy because of the skepticism attached to the practice. Therapeutic Touch will also be discussed later in this chapter.

Touch therapies, such as massage and Kangaroo Care, have long been successfully used in the growth and development of premature babies. Massage therapy, baby massage, or loving and caring touch (bonding), which are very popular today, are well documented by Auckett (1989). Not only can touch therapy help build a bond, but it can be used to calm crying, agitated, and unsettled babies.

MASSAGE THERAPY

Massage therapy, also called *therapeutic massage,* has been used for centuries to create balance and restore a sense of well-being by increasing blood flow throughout the body (Ginton, 1997). This, in turn, increases the oxygen-carrying potential of the body and the flow of lymph, thereby increasing the removal of toxins. According to Greene (1997), massage therapy is a "drugless" therapy that has been known to relieve headaches, insomnia, digestive disorders, arthritis, asthma, carpel tunnel syndrome, sinusitis, and minor aches and pains.

As previously stated, massage therapy involves using the hands to directly apply

pressure and motion to the skin and underlying muscle of a client for the purposes of physical and psychological relaxation, improvement of circulation, relief of sore muscles, and other therapeutic purposes. *Lexicon Webster English Dictionary* (1978) defines "massage" as the act or art of treating the body by rubbing or kneading to stimulate circulation or increase suppleness. The techniques of massage therapy include stroking, kneading, tapping, compression, vibration, rocking, and friction. Massage therapy may involve the use of oils, lotions, powders, and other lubricants. It may also be used in conjunction with aromatherapy (Huebscher & Shuler, 2003; Keegan, 1998).

History of Massage Therapy

The healing powers of massage have a long history. In the 5th century B.C., the Greek physician Hippocrates wrote about the experience of rubbing to loosen joints that are too rigid. Although different cultures, including the Chinese, Egyptians, and Romans, have employed different techniques and types of massage, the techniques used today in the United States were not introduced until the late 19th century, when Per Henrik Ling, a Swedish gymnast, formulated the principle of the popular Swedish massage after a visit to China. Before Swedish massage became popular, the ancient Chinese, Egyptians, and Romans had employed different massage techniques. Massage therapy is practiced in many professions, such as sports medicine, chiropractics, Chinese medicine, and ayurveda, and can be performed in conjunction with many other types of complementary and alternative medicine (CAM).

Therapeutic massage is also not new to the practice of nursing. The types of massage commonly used by nurses as interventions since the beginning of nursing are back rubs and foot massage. According to Dossey et al. (2000), back care is a common practice used especially by diploma-prepared nurses and it has always been incorporated into the standard morning bathing and evening care routines in most hospitals. As noted by Huebscher and Shuler (2003), today's health care system is so driven by conventional health care practices and medicines that many NAC therapies have fallen by the wayside. Their book provides a much-needed in-depth plan for the use of holistic NAC modalities, including massage, for the management of many, if not all, illnesses.

Techniques and Types of Massage Therapy

There are approximately one hundred different types of massage and bodywork techniques practiced today (University of Maryland Medical Center [UMM], 2013). Various forms of massage have been applied by different cultures (Kuhn, 1999). Although Swedish massage is the most popular type of massage therapy today, various techniques used by different cultures has led to the many different types of massages that exist today. Table 9-1 lists some of the well-known types of massage therapy.

Swedish massage incorporates classical massage techniques with those used in other types of massage therapy (Field, 2000; Kuhn, 1999). The basic strokes used in Swedish massage are:

- effleurage – light stroking or touching that is focused horizontally
- petrissage – kneading with a vertical lift technique
- friction (rubbing) – quick, short movements of the hand and fingertips over superficial tissues transversely
- percussion (tapotement) – the application of downward vertical pressure with abrupt release, including tapping, slapping, cupping, and beating
- vibration or shaking – pressing down and then back and forth in a particular place.

TABLE 9-1: EXAMPLES OF MASSAGE THERAPIES

- Reflexology (hand and foot)
- Rolfing
- Shiatsu
- Deep tissue massage
- Traditional European massage
- Contemporary Western massage
- Swedish massage
- Oriental massage
- Sports massage
- Acupressure
- Chair-seated massage
- Infant or baby massage
- Lomi lomi
- Gigong
- African massage
- Manual lymph drainage
- Hot stone massage

Benefits of Massage Therapy

Massage therapy has several holistic benefits. Metabolically, massage can prepare muscles and soft tissue for exercise as well as recovery from the effects of exercise activity. Psychologically, massage can reduce tension, anger, fear, fatigue, depression, anxiety, and confusion. Massage has been shown to reduce anxiety and lower stress hormones, and it is one of the most widely used relaxation modalities (Greene, 2000).

The main goal of massage therapy is to encourage healing by promoting the flow of blood and lymph, relieving tension, stimulating nerves, and stretching and loosening muscles and connective tissues to help keep them elastic. Massage techniques vary depending on the type of massage being performed. However, most types of massage include the use of soothing agents, such as oils or lotions; rubbing strokes; effleurage; petrissage; and tapotement.

According to Bright (2002), massage employs mechanical methods that directly affect the nervous system, chemical system, and the endocrine system. Manual techniques, such as pressing, pulling, rubbing, staccato, light touch, and deep tissue massage, are used to produce the desired effects. The increased circulation that results helps to flush body wastes, such as lactic acid, thereby restoring flexibility and range of motion.

According to Keegan (1998) and Huebscher and Shuler (2003), research has shown that massage can be used for a wide range of clinical conditions, including arthritis, high blood pressure, stress management, dementia, eating disorders, asthma, allergies, fibromyalgia, menopause, and sleep disorders as well as for smoking cessation.

Related Professional Issues

Certification and Licensure

According to the Commission on Massage Training Accreditation (COMTA), potential massage therapists must choose a licensed and accredited school for their education. They must also undergo hundreds of hours of class and practice to become certified and are required to follow COMTA standards of practice.

Although anyone can perform back rubs, to become a massage therapist, one has to complete a hands-on practice in one of the many massage schools located throughout the United States. Licensure varies from state to state. Certification is required to practice as a massage therapist. Naturalhealers.com provides a list of massage schools in the United States.

Contraindications

Massage therapy can provide welcome relief from the many symptoms caused by daily stress and activity. However, it is important to remember that massage therapy is not recommended for everyone and it can involve risk in certain circumstances. Massage therapy is also not a cure for any serious or life-threatening medical disorder. According to Huebscher and Shuler (2003) and Rankin-Box (2001), massage therapy is contraindicated in clients with acute illness or injury, fever, recent surgery, cardiovascular or respiratory insufficiency, and some psychological conditions. Before using any massage therapy agent, practitioners should ask about allergies or sensitivity to the product. Massage should not be performed over varicose veins, suspected or known phlebitis, deep vein thrombosis, skin lesions, or fractures and should not be performed in the presence of an open wound.

THERAPEUTIC TOUCH

History of Therapeutic Touch

In 1972, Dolores Krieger, a doctoral degree nursing student, and Dora Kunz, a natural healer, developed a new and controversial therapy called Therapeutic Touch. Like other touch therapies, the practice was derived from several ancient healing practices, including the old tradition of "laying on of the hands." Krieger formally introduced Therapeutic Touch to the nursing community in 1975 in a publication in the *American Journal of Nursing*.

According to Hawk (2000), Therapeutic Touch is the relearning or resurgence of ancient healing techniques that offer a holistic approach to healing. Krieger (1998), now a professor at New York University, continues to explore and expand the possibilities of Therapeutic Touch as she actively travels the world to share her knowledge and experience.

Therapeutic Touch is now being taught not only to nurses but also to professionals in other disciplines in the United States. Although it originally had to overcome much skepticism, Hawk (2000) notes that, in Canada, Therapeutic

Touch has grown rapidly and received positive feedback from patients. In Canadian hospitals, Therapeutic Touch is now used in oncology and maternity wards, with organ transplants, in intensive care units, and in other wards. Most Canadian nurses learn this skill on a voluntary basis. Hawk, who cofounded The Therapeutic Touch Network of Ontario, has assisted in organizing similar organizations in Alberta, the Atlantic Provinces, British Columbia, Manitoba, and Quebec (Hawk, 2000).

Description

Therapeutic Touch is not a religion, but the practice has roots in ancient shamanism. Physical contact is not necessary with Therapeutic Touch; however, some practitioners combine the practice with other NAC therapies, such as hypnosis, massage, acupressure, and counseling some of which do involve touch.

The practice of Therapeutic Touch as a holistic alternative and complementary therapy is really a contemporary interpretation of several ancient healing practices founded on the premise that the body, mind, emotion, and spirit form a complex dynamic energy field. In Therapeutic Touch, all healing is self-healing and the practitioner is primarily a facilitator. According to Newshan and Schuller-Civitella (2003), Therapeutic Touch is effective for promoting emotional and spiritual healing and stimulating the body's natural recuperative and healing processes.

Unlike massage therapy, which basically involves manipulation of the muscles and soft tissue, Therapeutic Touch is based on the idea that energy radiates through and around our bodies, and that illness and injury are the results of depleted or unbalanced flows in that energy. The practice of Therapeutic Touch is the process whereby the practitioner consciously uses his or her hands to direct and focus energy to stimulate and enhance the patient's own natural healing energies. According to Hawk (2000) and Krieger (1979, 1998), Therapeutic Touch is also based on the quantum theories of the universe being made up of energy fields and, therefore, the phenomenon cannot be observed.

Of all the different types of CAM and NAC therapies used today, Therapeutic Touch is one modality that is easy for skeptics to challenge as "science." This is because outcomes can usually only be measured subjectively by "feeling," which makes the practice difficult to scientifically study. Many skeptics, therefore, call Therapeutic Touch a pseudoscience, amoral or anti-Christian, a cult practice, Wiccan, a reconstruction of ancient Celtic Pagan religions, voodoo science, or a paranormal or religious activity masquerading as science. The majority of skeptics claim that, because Therapeutic Touch involves rechanneling and transfer of energy, it may be attracting demonic spirits from the spirit world (Robinson, 2003).

In Therapeutic Touch, centering is a very critical step. Centering is a sense of self-relatedness that involves concentration of thought in a place of inner being, a place of quietude within oneself where one can feel truly integrated, unified, and focused.

In order to understand how the universe operates, we must be open to understanding the concept of energy discussed in previous chapters. It also requires a change in paradigm from the mechanistic, Newtonian model of the universe to the new Einsteinian paradigm, philosophy, and science also discussed previously. In this new paradigm, as in many ancient cultures, illness is viewed as an interruption of the flow of energy in the body. The goal, therefore, in healing and promoting wholeness (holism) is to rebalance energy flow. However, as society evolves and continues to embrace the Newtonian perspective, the ability of humans to interconnect with nature has been denigrated and devalued. Today, stressors are part of our lives and we live with stress on an ongoing basis. The revisitation of therapies such as Therapeutic Touch can help us to better appreciate our potential for self-healing and to appreciate the concept of energy in healing.

Like the new theories of interconnectedness, Therapeutic Touch is grounded in the concept of wholeness. The theory behind the effectiveness of Therapeutic Touch now includes Martha Rogers' theory of Unitarian Energy Field (Rankin-Box, 2001).

Four Steps of Therapeutic Touch

The practice of Therapeutic Touch involves gentle manipulation of the body's energy flow as a whole and includes four basic steps: centering, assessment, intervention, and evaluation/closure.

(1) Centering – the therapist becomes "centered" by using breathing, imagery, and meditation to achieve an altered state of consciousness for their self.

(2) Assessment – the therapist holds their hands 2-4 inches away from the client assessing the energy field from head to toe and from back to front by placing the hands close to the client with palms open. The objective of this step is to get as much information about the client's energy field as possible. Therapists often describe feelings of warmth, coolness, static, and tingling over the areas of energy "congestion" or "blockage."

(3) Intervention – once the therapist locates a congested or blocked area, they will move their hands in a repetitive rhythmic motion, starting at the top of the blocked area and moving down and away from the body. This action, known as unruffling is a step in which the client's energy field is being smoothed, and is repeated until the thera-

pist no longer senses congestion or until the client begins to feel relief. The therapist will also visualize and transmit life energy to specific areas of the client's body, also intended to correct imbalances.

(4) Evaluation/Closure – once the client has had a few minutes to relax, the therapist will then ask how he or she feels. The therapist may recheck the energy field to be certain no blockages were overlooked (UMM, 2013).

As a noninvasive healing tool, the main functions of Therapeutic Touch are relaxation and pain reduction. This touch therapy has been proven to decrease stress and anxiety, reduce pain and insomnia, ease breathing, and accelerate wound healing (Rankin-Box, 2001). It is also used to treat headaches, chronic pain, and burns (Spence & Olson, 1997).

Related Professional Issues

Certification

Anyone can be trained to become a Therapeutic Touch practitioner and anyone can try Therapeutic Touch. To become a Therapeutic Touch practitioner, potential students must attend a 12-hour or longer workshop in which the basic concepts of Therapeutic Touch are taught. After that, a 1-year mentorship with a qualified Therapeutic Touch practitioner is required. To acquire Therapeutic Touch certification, the student must then complete intermediate and advanced level workshops. Teachers of Therapeutic Touch should practice Therapeutic Touch regularly, at least two times per week for 5 years, and undergo 1 year of teaching mentorship with a qualified Therapeutic Touch teacher.

Precautions, Risks, and Contraindications

Therapeutic Touch should not be practiced or entered into lightly because it involves energy transfer or rechanneling. Before performing Therapeutic Touch, practitioners should tell clients to alert them if they feel dizzy or uncomfortable at any time during the therapy. It is important to remember that Therapeutic Touch is a "no touch" therapeutic modality and, as such, the practitioner should be careful not to get his or her hands too close to certain body parts, such as the head, to prevent uneven flow of energy. Clients with a history of physical or sexual abuse should have clear expectations about the process, so that there are no misconceptions or fears (UMM, 2013). Although Therapeutic Touch can be used on pregnant women, it should be done only by experienced practitioners because it involves a complex set of energy fields from both the mother and fetus (Mackereth & Wright, 1997). Therapeutic Touch is contraindicated for certain conditions such as individuals with fever or active inflammation (example: swollen, arthritic joint), as it may worsen those conditions; also, children, frail elders and very ill people should only be treated for a very short time. Some practitioners believe Therapeutic Touch should not be done on areas of the body where there is cancer (UMM, 2013).

It should be noted that Therapeutic Touch can be performed with other CAM or NAC therapeutics. In such cases, the practitioner must inform the client that Therapeutic Touch will be performed and explain that it is a no-contact form of "laying on of the hands."

Nursing and Therapeutic Touch

Therapeutic Touch is unique to nursing because this holistic practice grew up from and within the nursing profession (Fenton, 2003; Krieger, 1999). As nurses practice Therapeutic Touch at masters and doctoral programs, many are able to use it to connect theory and practice in appreciating healing. As a result, an extensive body of solid research has begun to emerge and research using Rogers' theory of energy field has provided some validity and support for this holistic nursing practice.

The American Nurses Association and the National League of Nursing support the teaching of Therapeutic Touch in several nursing schools across the country. Nurse Healers-Professional Associates International (NH-PAI), the official organization for Therapeutic Touch, has set forth standards, policies, procedures, ethical statements, and guidelines for teachers, mentors, and students practicing Therapeutic Touch.

Therapeutic Touch is usually employed as a complementary therapy rather than an alternative replacement for standard medical care, and it is recommended to be used with other types of CAM or NAC therapies. There is no licensing or formal Therapeutic Touch programs, but certificates are usually awarded to those who complete classes on Therapeutic Touch (Fenton, 2003; UMM, 2013). Although Therapeutic Touch is now a part of nursing practice, further research is needed to validate this holistic therapy and remove some of the stigmas associated with it.

CONCLUSION

Touch therapy encompasses a broad range of healing techniques, including massage therapy and Therapeutic Touch. Touch therapy is unique because the same touch can be interpreted differently in different cultures. According to Keegan (1998), Krieger (1998), and Spence and Olson (1997), millions of patients regularly seek out nontraditional NAC therapies, such as healing touch, massage, Therapeutic Touch, and other types of touch therapy because these therapies offer a holistic approach to healing. Nurses with proper training are in the position to administer any type of touch therapy in any clinical setting.

Anyone interested in learning some type of touch therapy should study the history, procedure, characteristics, cautions, safety and ethical issues, and responsibilities associated with the practice prior to using it. Touch therapy relies on a controlled environment, where sound, positioning, light, music, aroma, and other factors can be managed. Touch therapy can be enhanced with other CAM or NAC therapies, such as relaxation, guided imagery, music, and meditation.

ONLINE RESOURCES FOR TOUCH THERAPY

British Columbia Therapeutic Touch Network
    http://www.bctherapeutictouch.com

Nurse Healers: Professional Associates International
    http://www.therapeutic-touch.org

Healing Touch International, Inc.
    http://www.healingtouch.net

Quantum Touch: Energy Healing
    http://www.quantumtouch.com

Holistic Energy Healing
    http://www.holisticmed.com/www/energy.
    html

EXAM QUESTIONS

CHAPTER 9
Questions 62–71

Note: Choose the one option that BEST answers each question.

62. Examples of touch therapy include massage therapy, Therapeutic Touch, reflexology, and

    a. acupuncture.
    b. herbal therapy.
    c. music therapy.
    d. shiatzu.

63. The act or art of treating the body by rubbing or kneading to stimulate circulation or increase suppleness is known as

    a. Healing Touch.
    b. Kangaroo Care.
    c. massage.
    d. Therapeutic Touch.

64. Massage therapy has been used for centuries for a number of therapeutic and medical benefits. In nursing, the most common type of therapeutic massage is

    a. foot care.
    b. back rub.
    c. spine massage.
    d. temple massage.

65. The most popular type of massage therapy is

    a. reflexology.
    b. shiatsu.
    c. Swedish massage.
    d. oriental massage.

66. Before performing massage therapy, the nurse should check the client's

    a. pulse rate.
    b. blood pressure.
    c. body mass index.
    d. allergies.

67. The nurse who developed Therapeutic Touch is

    a. Jean Watson.
    b. Dolores Krieger.
    c. Florence Nightingale.
    d. Dorothy Orem.

68. The most recent theory of wholeness and interconnectedness that guides the practice of Therapeutic Touch is the theory of

    a. chakras.
    b. meridian pressure points.
    c. Unitarian Energy Fields.
    d. Newton.

69. In Therapeutic Touch, the step in which the client's energy field is being smoothed to keep energy flowing in a natural pattern is referred to as

    a. assessment.
    b. centering.
    c. unruffling.
    d. unroofing.

continued on next page

70. As a noninvasive healing tool, the main therapeutic function of Therapeutic Touch is

    a. diet management.

    b. treatment of stomach ulcers.

    c. relief of menopause symptoms.

    d. relaxation and pain reduction.

71. When performing Therapeutic Touch, caution should be taken to avoid the

    a. liver.

    b. stomach.

    c. tail bone.

    d. head.

CHAPTER 10

FOLK HEALING THERAPIES AND PRACTICES

CHAPTER OBJECTIVE

Upon completion of this chapter, the learner will be able to describe the history and practice of folk healing and its uses as a holistic alternative and complementary therapy.

LEARNING OBJECTIVES

After studying this chapter, the learner will be able to:

1. Describe the meaning of folk healing practices or therapeutics.
2. Discuss the history and characteristics of African healing practices.
3. Define African folk healing as a holistic and complementary therapeutic modality.
4. List different types of African healing therapies and their holistic benefits as alternative and complementary therapies.
5. Differentiate between herbalistic, homeopathic and spiritual healing.
6. Describe the history and beliefs of Chinese medicine.
7. Identify at least three types of Chinese medicine.
8. Recognize the benefits and risks of acupuncture and other forms of Chinese medicine.

INTRODUCTION

Folk healing is a practice common to every culture. Since the beginning of civilization, leaders in every culture sought natural ways to heal the members of their communities.

However, with the coming of the scientific age, many of the ancient folk healing practices have been revised, adapted, renamed, and improved. From the Chinese use of acupuncture to Indian ayurveda and African faith and symbolic healing, all folk healing practices have something in common: the use of plants and energy. Estimates of fold healing practices range from 85% in countries such as Africa to approximately 5% in the United States and include homeopathy and plant based remedies (Frass et al., 2012). According to DuToit (1998), the World Health Organization (WHO) there are many of the world's population that rely on medicines derived from plants for their primary health care – that is four out of every five individuals in the world. This includes the United States because, as discussed in Chapter 4, many drugs manufactured today originated from herbs.

According to the Lock et al. (2001); Mbiti (1990); McHenry (1998); Ulett, Han, & Han (1998); and Vontress (1999), folk healing practices are a major part of the primary health care and healing practices of many cultures. Although there is currently a shift toward primary health care in certain countries, the economic situation in many other countries has made it practically impossible to achieve the goal of primary health care for all citizens.

Simply stated, folk healing refers to the healing practices of a particular culture. Although the public and modern health care system have recognized the folk healing practices of some cultures (for example, Chinese acupuncture and Japanese tai chi), many African folk healing practices go unrecognized and unacknowledged. Although the work of the Egyptians has been widely acclaimed, Egypt is only one of the forty-four African countries. Some other African countries share health care practices with the Egyptians but continue to go unrecognized. The purpose of this chapter, therefore, is to present the folk healing practices used specifically by the African and Chinese cultures.

AFRICAN FOLK HEALING PRACTICES

History and Description

Africans have been noted to be the root of human civilization. In fact, Lock et al. (2001) note that some of the earliest evidence of medical practices comes from Africa. To understand the health care practices of Africans, it is important to have an appreciation of the size of the continent of Africa. It is a large continent that comprises a kaleidoscope of countries and cultures with a rich history of vast and diverse traditions. However, most African cultures share some similarities. One such similarity is that traditional and natural healing modalities have been and still are a major aspect of the health care practices. As of 2005, there were forty-four African countries. Egypt, a country that occupies the northeast corner of Africa and one of the most popular nations, has documented traditional health care and healing practices since the beginning of civilization and is currently known for its practice of aromatherapy, massage, and music therapies among others (Bright, 2002; Buckle, 2001; Kozier, Erb, Berman, & Burke, 2000; Mentgen, 2001; Rankin-Box, 2001).

Most African societies are still male-dominated, polygamous, and characterized by diverse ethnic and cultural beliefs and many different languages. The cultural belief systems continue to dictate African health care and healing practices. Traditional health practices are closely linked with religious and cultural traditions. Today, traditional healers and therapies coexist with modern medicine (biomedicine). Since African countries are still developing and the majority of citizens are very poor, many African citizens cannot afford modern health care. In addition, after building hospital and clinic infrastructures, many countries found that they could not afford medical equipment and supplies or even their health care providers. Therefore, the predominant health care practice of most Africans still involves folk healers, native doctors, or cultural, magical, and religious ethnic healers. Vontress (1999) claims that African folk healing involves making diagnoses that are unscientific and religion-based and interventions that are psychological, spiritual, and physical. For example, dance and music are sometimes used as part of African folk healing practices.

Traditional African health care practices are ancient but have evolved in the last two centuries. The recent interest in complementary and alternative medicine (CAM) and natural, alternative, and complementary (NAC) therapies (Morrison & Thornton, 1999; Stone, 2001) has led some university scientists and doctors in Africa to study the art and science of native doctors and traditional healers (Chipfakacha, 1997; Cocks & Dold, 2000; Homsy et al., 1999). This renewed interest is like Homer's *Odyssey*. However, unlike Odysseus's Greek mythological adventurous journey home that took years, CAM therapy is a journey that can be found immediately in the stories of early traditional or folk healers, such as the Egyptians and other African cultures.

The Egyptians are well-known for having advanced knowledge of medicine more than

5,000 years ago. Unlike the Chinese culture, in which the majority of practices were written down (Bright, 2002), most African medicines (other than Egyptian) were transmitted to other cultures and generations via oral history.

Vontress (1999) notes that the ravages of poverty, drought, and disease, along with a fragmented health care system, have resulted in the continued use of African folk healers who include rituals in their traditional healing practices. However, African folk healers are erroneously referred to as *shamans* or *shamanic practitioners*. Rather, these practitioners should be viewed as herbalistic, spiritual, and ritualistic healers.

African Folk Healing Beliefs and Practices

Cultural and spiritual factors and practices influence the concept of illness in Africa. Folk healers in Africa have special areas of expertise. Folk therapies or remedies include variations of massage, or plant remedies, and dermabrasive practices, such as cupping, pinching, rubbing, and burning. Dermabrasive therapies and practices are believed to restore health by releasing "bad energy" or "evil spirits." Amulets that can be worn on a bracelet or necklace or pinned to clothing are believed to provide some protection against evil spirits and certain illnesses. For example, amulets inscribed with verses of the Koran or the Bible and decorated with turquoise stones or charms on the hand or fingers are used to enhance protective powers or energy against the "evil eye." Strings around the neck, ankles, and waist are also worn to prevent harm.

In many African countries, specifically in South Africa, folk medicine has been integrated with elements from traditional Africans and immigrant Europeans (Du Toit, 1998). Lock et al. (2001) note that, since the colonial and missionary eras of African history,

the mixing of Islamic and Christian religions with African traditional folk healing practices has formed a new medico-religious practice called *syncretic faith healing*. This has led to the creation of churches such as the celestial churches, which are well known for helping with the healing of illnesses, particularly mental illness. Dance therapy, prayers, holy water, and imagery are among some of the NAC health care therapies used in Africa (Morrison & Thornton, 1999; Vontress, 1999; Wilkinson, Gcabashe, & Lurie, 1999).

African healing and health care practices are sometimes regarded as inflexible, unchanging, voodooistic, mystical, and magical, but their role and impact on the global health care system and healing cannot be underestimated. Many African countries have roots in the traditions of their ancient cultures, and these traditions are passed down from generation to generation or are learned or acquired as a spiritual encounter or calling. Like traditional healers of any culture, African healers are often powerful men or women with strong celestial, spiritual, and magical powers (Tsey, 1997). Many traditional healers claim to have the ability to communicate with a higher being, such as God or Allah. Such powers are used to either save an entire community, as in the case of "town criers," or used to treat simple or complex physical and mental illnesses, stress, and injuries.

Natural and supernatural beliefs and forces still hold a strong place in the traditional health care practices of Africans. Traditional healers often seek consultation with a priest or God to find luck or avoid evil and illness. Furthermore, some illnesses are perceived to originate from supernatural, magical, or religious beliefs and, therefore, must be cured by traditional treatments or magical spells. As in the past, people still believe in the practice of sorcery and take daily precautions or make periodic sacrifices to protect themselves and their families from harm, jealousy, and evil spirits (Vontress, 1999).

A strong belief in supernatural powers or a supreme being also still exists. Christian, Islamic, and pagan practices, such as prayer, verses, amulets, and the art of appealing to different icons, spirits, or gods, are among the beliefs central to African health care practices. Some of the general beliefs and assumptions underlying traditional African health care practices are presented in Table 10-1.

TABLE 10-1: TRADITIONAL AFRICAN HEALTH CARE BELIEFS

- Human beings have two parts: body (mass) and spirit.
- The mind is a part of the spirit that makes the whole (holistic) person.
- Spiritual and cultural beliefs are important for healing the body, mind, spirit and for total (holistic) well-being.
- Health care is a mix of biomedical, magical, spiritual, traditional, holistic, and supernatural beliefs and practices.
- Modern medicine has its roots in the practices of traditional and herbal healers.
- Roots, trees, herbs, plants, flowers, and seeds are the tools of traditional healers from which medicines are made.
- Traditional healers are like facilitators who assist people to rebalance energy from illness to wellness.
- Supernatural forces, spiritual powers, and the notion of hot and cold energy are the roots of traditional practices.

Despite the shift toward primary health care, the grim economical situation in many African countries makes it practically impossible to implement. Some very rural areas with limited access to biomedicine still favor traditional or folk practices and spiritual healers over Western medicine. In many African countries today, there are still more traditional and faith healers than Western healers. As a whole, Africans continue to practice holistic therapies and use preventive healing practices (Popoola, 2004, as cited in Huebscher & Shuler, 2003).

Holistic and Preventive Practices

Holistic therapy and preventive health care practices are part of traditional African health care systems. These practices include a combination of self-care, herbal medicines, and religious arts. Other health care practices include touch therapy, such as therapeutic body massage, foot massage, and acupressure; food therapy and rituals such as garlic and onions hung in the home or on the body to drive out evil spirits and used in cooking to prevent illness; "magic hand" for healing, bone setting, and pain management; and traditional dance and drumming (Vontress, 1999).

Types of African Folk Healing Practices and Their Benefits

African traditional or folk healers use many types of therapies in their practice. These include ancient healing practices or native doctors, herbal healing practices, healing remedies (massage, chiropractic), dermabrasive (cupping, pinching, rubbing, burning), amulets, prayers, holy water, ashes, rituals (birth and death practices), healing dance, town criers, magic hands and other touch practices, and a combination of home remedies. Folk healers also include many respected and skilled bonesetters, who are well known throughout the rural and urban parts of different African countries and are famous for their orthopedic and wound-healing skills. Folk healers or native doctors treat sprains, swellings, and other physical and mental illnesses. They also are counselors who give advice and use healing cultural artifacts and icons, such as stones, beads, and roots (Vontress, 1999). Some specific NAC therapeutic practices used by Africans are presented and discussed in the rest of this section.

Herbalism and Homeopathy

Herbalists are folk healers who are skilled in the use of herbs, roots, and plants. Homeopaths are local chemists or pharmacists who mix extracts from roots and plants for medicinal purposes and also create teas. However, herbs are not the only healing tools used by herbalists and homeopaths. They also promote self-care and self-medication. Herbalists treat common disorders and also specialize in the treatment of the "evil eye." The evil eye is believed to cast spells or curses that could lead to illness and death. This belief cuts across many African countries. Herbalists and homeopaths often boil ingredients and roots into teas or steam inhalants. Such steam inhalants are frequently used as bronchodilators. This type of treatment is similar to those used by respiratory therapists in Western cultures today.

Homeopathic practice is strongly rooted in the belief that the body has the capacity to heal itself. Unlike conventional medicine, which focuses on suppressing bodily responses, replacing substances that the body has failed to produce, or using small doses of a disease-producing agent to sensitize or desensitize the immune system, homeopathic medicine or remedies initiate the body's return to balance (homeostatic mechanism). Homeopathic remedies or medicines are usually manufactured from natural substances, such as plants, metals, minerals, venoms, animals, and bacteria. A commonly used remedy is the extract of the plant belladonna (deadly nightshade) for treatment of fever and pain.

Spiritual, Faith, and Imaginary Healers

Spiritual, faith, and imaginary healing has to do with the relationship of the mind and spirit to the body. Prophets of celestial or syncretic churches are classified as traditional healers or shamans. However, spiritual, faith, and imaginary healers have their roots in ancient spiritual practices as well as in Christian churches. In some religious practices, such as Islam, which dictates health promotion practices, citizens take a passive role. In Christianity, prayers and the healing power of God are used for protection against misfortune, and holy water is used as a symbol of communion with the healer. Christian healing churches, such as the Celestial, "Aladura," or faith healing churches, are common in Africa.

Today, most African countries have more churches that claim to help with the healing of physical and mental illnesses than they have schools or hospitals. Drumming, dance therapy, prayers, holy water, and imagery are among the NAC therapies used in Africa as part of faith healing (Morrison & Thornton, 1999; Wilkinson, Gcabashe, & Lurie, 1999). Spiritual healing is usually done by praying for or with someone, by "laying on of the hands," by distance healing, and by symbolic rituals such as the cross or rosary. Personal prayers can instill hope and reduce the anxiety associated with many illnesses and stressors. Faith healing will be discussed in more detail in Chapter 11.

Symbolic Healing Rituals: Drumming and Coconuts

In almost every culture and tradition, symbolic rituals, such as drumming and dancing, are performed at festivities, celebrations, and spiritual events. However, these rituals can also be used in the process of trying to heal a person. Although the meaning of such activities varies from culture to culture, in African cultures, many of these activities are similar and have almost the same goal: to promote balance. They often serve as reminders that life is fragile, even in times of joy, and they can be used in times of trouble and stress to bring about peace.

Drumming, dancing, and birth rituals are among the spiritual healing rituals that are used in Africa. For example, many babies are still delivered at home with the mother squatting in a semiseated position or being tied to some object as a traditional healer chants and drums. Some traditional midwives still recommend the use of bellybands after delivery to assist with expulsion of the placenta and to decrease the size of the abdomen. In some African traditions, newborns are believed to be susceptible to evil influences during the first week of life, and caution is taken to limit the number and type of visitors who come close to the baby. Native midwives usually perform circumcision practices for male infants in the first 2 weeks of life. Mothers are usually instructed to drink only warm foods and liquids (Ogaga, 1999). Traditional practices and birth rituals also include numerous birth taboos which, if broken, are thought to affect the pregnancy and the newborn. Traditional birth attendants and midwives are often used for deliveries outside the hospital. Most African countries would not survive without the birth practices and skills of traditional midwives.

The coconut is often seen as a symbol for or metaphor of holism because of its vast uses for health and healing. When used in daily cooking, coconut oil can help protect from heart disease, cancer, and other degenerative conditions; improves digestion; strengthens the immune system; and helps with weight loss. Much of the research on the nutritional and medicinal benefits of coconut oil has been done by Dr. Mary Enig, who classified the coconut as a "functional food" (Enig, 1999). She has specifically identified lauric acid as a key ingredient in coconut products and noted that approximately 50% of the fatty acids in coconut fat are lauric

acid. Lauric acid is a medium-chain fatty acid that has the additional benefit of being formed into monolaurin in the human or animal body (Organic Facts, 2014). Monolaurin is an antiviral, antibacterial, and antiprotozoal monoglyceride used by humans and animals to destroy lipid-coated viruses, such as human immunodeficiency virus (HIV), herpes, and influenza, and various other pathogenic bacteria, including *Helicobacter pylori* and various protozoa (Enig, 1999; Fife, 1999; Jones, 1997).

As a "functional food," coconut is now being recognized by the medical community as a powerful tool against many diseases. According to Fife (2000), a naturopathic doctor and the author of the book *The Healing Miracles of Coconut Oil,* coconut oil is the healthiest oil on earth. Research is also currently being done on the incredible nutritional value of pure coconut oil. Once wrongly accused of increasing cholesterol levels, coconut oil is now used by doctors in the treatment of various disorders. Studies conducted in the Philippines, the Caribbean, Malaysia, the South Pacific, New Zealand, Asia, and the United States have shown the health benefits of the coconut and its oil. The coconut is also a major part of African, Asian, and Caribbean diets (Fife, 1999). Furthermore, Huebscher and Shuler (2003) note that the coconut is a critical part of diet therapy in Indian ayurveda.

Practical Application of African Healing Practices

Other than herbal and faith healing practices, the majority of African folk healing practices are not well recognized. Reasons include a lack of funds to research and archive the practices and the sovereignty and lack of cooperation among African countries. Unlike Chinese medicine, which has been able to spread and penetrate other cultures, including Japan, Europe, and America, African healing practices are still finding their place in the modern world. In Africa, however, the majority of African healers are well respected and trusted as holistic healers (Vontress, 1999). African healing practices, such as herbal therapy and spiritual or faith healing, should be used as complements rather than alternatives.

CHINESE MEDICINE

Description

Like African folk healing, traditional Chinese medicine is a holistic therapeutic that is a combination of therapies. According to Rankin-Box (2001), Chinese medicine includes **massage therapy, herbalism, and acupuncture.** These various therapeutic modalities can be practiced separately or in combination. Also like African health care practices, prevention and self-healing are key components of Chinese medicine. Meditation, dietary regulation, body works, and the principle of Tao (or Dao, or leader) are also part of Chinese healing practices (NIH, 2013).

Diet and herbal therapy are widely used in Chinese medicine. The use of chi, energies, body meridians, organs, and yin and yang (see Figure 10-1) are also common in Chinese medicine. Treatment with Chinese medicine depends on knowledge of complex philosophical laws that govern the relationship between yin and yang. In Chinese medicine, yin and yang are the base for symptomatic diagnosis and the use of herbal therapy. Yin indicates coolness, and yang indicates heat. In addition to the use of yin and yang, the Chinese use four methods to determine problems or make diagnoses: observation, inquiry, listening, and palpation. Chinese medical texts have guidelines on how to examine patients (Zhang, Bausell, Lao, Handwerger, & Berman, 2003). Another important aspect of Chinese medicine is that their medicines are

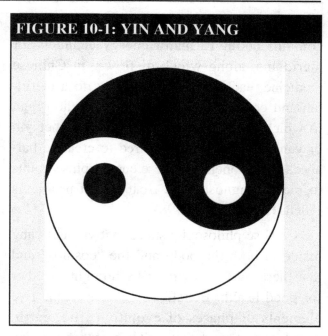

FIGURE 10-1: YIN AND YANG

generally made naturally from herbs. According to Zhang, Bausell, Lao, Handwerger, and Berman (2003), traditional Chinese medicine differs from Western medicine in the sense that treatment is highly individualized and the practitioner relies heavily on clinical experience and subjective observations and palpation.

Traditional Chinese Medicine Beliefs

Although thousands of years old, Chinese medicine is now becoming very popular and well-respected in places outside of China. The National Center for Complementary and Alternative Medicine recognizes and classifies many alternative medical practices from other cultures as indigenous healing practices; however, Chinese medicine has been given more attention and scientific focus. It is now being openly used in place of or in combination with Western medicine. The practice is still heavily based on ancient ideas and beliefs surrounding the use of herbs, yin and yang, acupuncture, and massage.

According to McCaffrey and Fowler (2003), Chinese medicine is based on and uses a network of channels and reservoirs that transfer, transform, move, and store qi. Qi flows through channels and reservoirs that are like the wires of an electrical circuit. The body contains about 12 major energy channels, or meridians, along which qi flows. In Chinese medicine, each organ is connected to a meridian and each meridian is named for the organ to which it connects. Each organ is either yin or yang, and organs are paired to create a balance. Practitioners use these energy pulse points to make diagnoses and treat health problems (Ulett, Han, & Han, 1998).

Chinese philosophy states that yin and yang reside in both the body and the "cosmos" and that these two forces must be brought together for good health. Beliefs also center on the five elements or phases of evolution: fire, earth, metal, wood, and water. Those who practice traditional Chinese medicines believe that there are five main centers in the human body: heart/mind, lungs, liver, spleen, and kidneys. Six external disease-causing factors also exist: winds, cold, heat, moisture, dryness, and fire. The Chinese also believe that our bodies are guided or influenced by seven emotions: happiness, anger, worry, pensiveness, grief, fear, and surprise. These belief systems and assumptions have driven the practice of Chinese medicine for centuries (see Table 10-2).

Types of Chinese Medicine

In **Chinese herbal medicine,** cold or cool herbs are used to treat hot or yang illnesses or problems, whereas hot or warm herbs are used to treat cold or yin illnesses or problems. Herbs can also be classified as heaven, or upper-class herbs; man, or middle--class herbs; and earth, or lower-class herbs. Other ways to classify are in terms of their relationship to blood, energy (chi), meridians, organs, and yin and yang. The Chinese use a wide variety of herbs, some of which are herbs used by other cultures, including ginseng, cinnamon, garlic, ginger, and cayenne pepper (Zhang, Bausell, Lao, Handwerger, & Berman, 2003).

TABLE 10-2: TRADITIONAL CHINESE MEDICINE BELIEFS

- The human body is an organic whole.
- The human body has an inseparable connection with the natural world and the universe as a whole.
- Everyone is born with self-healing abilities.
- Destructive energy patterns, such as cancer, can be interrupted and broken.
- The body has the ability to regenerate its immune system.
- The best medicine is prevention.
- There are six external disease-causing factors: winds, cold, heat, moisture, dryness, and fire.
- Seven emotions influence health: happiness, anger, worry, pensiveness, grief, fear, and surprise.

Acupuncture is the practice of inserting needles into specific exterior body locations (called *acupoints*). It is used to relieve pain, induce surgical anesthesia, and achieve other therapeutic purposes. Acupuncture should not be confused with **acupressure**, which is a type of touch therapy that is more like massage of pressure or pulse points in which no needles are used. In acupuncture, specially shaped needles that are round or blunt, three-edged, sword-like, sharp, and round or filiform are used to balance body energy. According to Carlsson (2002), the word *acupuncture* comes from two root words, *acus* meaning sharp and *pungere* meaning to puncture. In addition to needle piercing, acupuncture practitioners use heat, pressure, friction, suction, and electromagnetic energy to stimulate energy (chi) for the purpose of restoring health (Ovechkin, Lee, & Kim, 2001). According to Dung (1995), the body has about 365 acupuncture points that are connected by meridians.

In Chinese, the word "massage," or *amma*, means to calm with the hand. Like acupuncture, **Chinese massage** aims to break up the blockage of energy flow through the meridians. Some of the techniques used in Chinese massage are light pressure, rubbing, kneading, pressing, vibration, tapping, and circulating pressure. As mentioned in Chapter 9, these techniques have been adopted into the practices of Swedish massage as well as into other types of massage therapy.

Benefits of Chinese Medicine: Acupuncture

According to Ulett, Han, and Han (1998), acupuncture has been found to be helpful in the relief of asthma, pain such as arthritis, migraines, depression, addictions such as heroin addiction, gastrointestinal disorders, and cardiovascular problems. Mann (2003) adds that reports have supported the use of acupuncture for many different types of pain, including back pain, dental and temporomandibular dysfunction, fibromyalgia, osteoarthritis, neck pain, and chronic pain (Cherkin, Sherman, Deyo, & Shekelle, 2003; Carlsson, 2002; McCaffrey & Fowler, 2003).

Although still controversial, millions of Americans use acupuncture yearly for chronic pain. Skeptics argue that acupuncture is just an elaborate placebo. In 2012, a more recent NCCAM-funded study regarding the effects of acupuncture on pain management, was published in the Archives of Internal Medicine. The study's evidence was based on two components: the patient's belief that the treatment would be effective i.e. the placebo effect; and the specific locations and depth of the acupuncture needles.

A group of researchers from the Acupuncture Trialists' Collaboration, reviewed data from high-quality randomized trials on acupuncture for chronic pain, and conducted a meta-analysis involving individual patient data from 17,922 people. The 29 high-quality randomized controlled trials investigated the use of acupuncture for back and neck pain, osteoarthritis, shoulder pain, or chronic headache. The trials used acupuncture vs simulated acupuncture (special effects that mimicked the real procedure), and acupuncture vs no-acupuncture controls.

The authors concluded that "the total effects of acupuncture, as experienced by patients in clinical practice, are clinically relevant. They also noted that their study provides the most robust evidence to date that acupuncture is more than just placebo and a reasonable referral option for patients with chronic pain" (NIH, 2014c).

Professional Issues Related to Chinese Medicine

Certification

Numerous schools and programs across the United States and around the world offer to teach and prepare candidates to practice Chinese medicine. These programs are between 4 and 5 years long and, at the end, award either a diploma or master's degree, depending on the scope of the program. Graduates of these programs may be called Qigong masters, Chinese physicians, or Taoist or Buddhist scholars (Crawford, Sparber, & Jonas, 2003; McCaffrey & Fowler, 2003). These programs are accredited by The Accreditation Commission for Acupuncture and Oriental Medicine (ACAOM) which is the national accrediting agency recognized by the U.S. Department of Education. The National Certification Commission for Acupuncture and Oriental Medicine (NCCAOM) is the only national organization that validates entry-level competency in the practice of acupuncture and Oriental medicine (AOM) through professional certification. Their websites are: ACAOM: http://www.acaom.org and NCCAOM: http://www.nccaom.org

The education and certification necessary to be able to perform acupuncture varies from state to state. Only a person fully trained in the practice of Chinese medicine can perform acupuncture. Nurses, however, can assist in assessment of the client after the procedure is performed and in properly educating a client before and after treatment.

Precautions, Risks, and Client Safety

The biggest risk associated with acupuncture treatment is the use of needles and the risk for infection and organ injury. Lao, Hamilton, Fu, and Berman (2003) conducted a comprehensive review of existing literature about the safety of the practice with mixed results. Despite this, the potential exists for transmission of infectious diseases, such as hepatitis, HIV, auricular infection, staphylococcal septicemia, spinal infection, and bacterial endocarditis. In addition, acupuncture also places clients at risk for pseudo-aneurysm, organ and tissue injuries, spinal cord injury, nerve injury, and other forms of tissue damage. Therefore, it is recommended that disposable needles be used in acupuncture (Mann, 2003) and that proper training and professional standards be followed (Lao, Hamilton, Fu, & Berman, 2003). Acupuncture is contraindicated with alcohol, large meals, hot baths, extreme emotional states and, in some cases, pregnancy (Rankin-Box, 2001).

CONCLUSION

Folk healing practices are common to every culture. In Africa, for instance, because of poverty and a lack of resources folk healing practices such as spiritual and faith healing, holistic and preventive practice, herbalism, homeopathy, supernatural belief, imaginative healers, and symbolic healing rituals are still a major part of health care. In Chinese medicine,

folk healing practices include the popular and well-known practice of acupuncture, Chinese herbs, and the Chinese holistic philosophy of yin and yang. Folk healing practices can be used to manage all kinds of current-day medical health problems.

ONLINE RESOURCES FOR FOLK HEALING

The Accreditation Commission for Acupuncture and Oriental Medicine (ACAOM)
http://www.acaom.org

American Association of Naturopathic Physicians
http://www.naturopathic.org

American Association of Acupuncture and Oriental Medicine
http://www.aaaomonline.org

The National Certification Commission for Acupuncture and Oriental Medicine (NCCAOM)
http://www.nccaom.org

The Transcendent Meditation Program
http://www.tm.org

The Universal healing Sanctuary
http://www.reikihealing.co.za

EXAM QUESTIONS

CHAPTER 10
Questions 72–78

Note: Choose the one option that BEST answers each question.

72. The country that occupies the northeast corner of Africa and has documented traditional health care and healing practices since the beginning of civilization is

    a. China.

    b. Sierra Leone.

    c. Egypt.

    d. Ivory Coast.

73. African folk healing practices are still heavily influenced by a belief in

    a. supernatural power.

    b. supernatural power and Tao.

    c. supernatural power and yang.

    d. yin and yang.

74. The therapeutic practice that is rooted in the belief that the body can heal itself and uses natural remedies is

    a. Chinese medicine.

    b. aromatherapy.

    c. herbal therapy.

    d. homeopathy.

75. In Chinese medicine, the philosophy of yin and yang is frequently associated with the concept of hot and cold. In this philosophy

    a. yin means chi.

    b. yang means chi.

    c. yin means hotness.

    d. yang mean hotness.

76. Channels or conduits through which energy flows or travels in the body are called

    a. qi.

    b. chakras.

    c. meridians.

    d. acupoints.

77. The use of touch in the manipulation of pressure points and meridians (in which no needles are used) is called

    a. acupuncture.

    b. acupressure.

    c. yoga.

    d. massage therapy.

78. In Chinese medicine, the word "amma" refers to

    a. acupressure.

    b. acupuncture.

    c. herbs.

    d. massage.

CHAPTER 11

SPIRITUAL HEALING PRACTICES

CHAPTER OBJECTIVE

Upon completion of this chapter, the learner will be able to discuss the history and practice of spiritual healing therapies, and their uses as holistic alternative and complementary therapies.

LEARNING OBJECTIVES

After studying this chapter, the reader will be able to:

1. Describe the history of spiritual healing practices.
2. Differentiate spiritual healing practices from prayer and other religious and shamanistic practices.
3. Describe spiritual healing practices as holistic complementary therapeutic modalities.
4. Specify the role of prayer as a spiritual healing practice.
5. Identify types of spiritual healing practices.
6. List the holistic benefits of spiritual healing practices as forms of alternative and complementary therapy.
7. Discuss the nursing responsibilities and implications associated with spiritual healing practices and prayer.

INTRODUCTION

The practice of spiritual healing is very common. Just like the use of other natural, alternative, and complementary (NAC) therapies, such as massage therapy and aromatherapy, the use of spiritual healing practices, especially prayer, and energy healing practices is also growing (Eisenberg et al., 1998). The practice of spiritual healing is not limited to any one religion. Spiritual healing can involve such activities as going to a church or mosque, worshipping an idol or a mountain, using prayer wheels (such as in Buddhism), visiting a hospital chapel, and meditating. It can also involve spiritual interventions, such as going to a group bible study or prayer group; reading the Bible, Koran, or other religious book; receiving pastoral visits in a hospital; confessing; and any other spiritual activity or intervention intended for the purpose of worshipping, fellowshipping with a group, or individual healing.

Spiritual healing practices can be found in every culture (Jonas & Crawford, 2003). These holistic practices allow devoted practitioners to transcend the ordinary world to a space where they are able to communicate with a higher being. Spiritual healing practices are sometimes examined in the same context as energy therapies, and the National Center for Complementary and Alternative Medicine (NCCAM) classifies these therapies together. However, the purpose of this chapter is primarily to discuss the practice of spiritual healing therapies, such as prayer, and relate their uses as holistic alternative and complementary therapies.

HISTORY AND CHARACTERISTICS OF SPIRITUAL HEALING PRACTICES

Spiritual healing practices are therapeutic healing practices that have been in existence since the beginning of civilization. They are a part of every culture's healing practices (Jonas & Crawford, 2003). These practices are holistic because they are designed to connect the body with the mind and spirit. In addition, spiritual healing practices allow devoted practitioners to transcend the ordinary world to a place where they are able to communicate with a higher being or power.

Spiritual healing is sometimes referred to as faith, energetic, mystical, and shamanic healing. However, shamanism is not simply spiritual healing. In many cultures, shamans are herbalists and community leaders that fulfill certain social and cultural nonhealth-related obligations. Although shamanism is not a religion, it is a form of spiritual tradition that addresses key elements, such as marriage, rites of passage, death and dying, and parenting. In many cultures, shamans operate based on a state of consciousness. They may also be called imaginative healers, voodooists, native doctors, wise men, priests, wiccans, witches and pagans, among other names. Some of these names have resulted in shamans being perceived in a negative light (Rankin-Box, 2001; Hung-Youn, 1999; Townsend, 2001).

Spiritual healing practices and religions are not one and the same. Every religion, however, has specific ways of practicing spiritual healing. The majority of the time, such practices are guided by the beliefs and assumptions of that particular religion, and not all citizens of a particular culture share the same religious beliefs. Spiritual healing practices can vary not only between cultures but also within them. Although many different religions and spiritual healing practices exist, the use of prayer is common to almost all religions and cultures. According to Ameling (2000), prayer is an ancient healing practice not generally available in the Western health care system. She notes that prayer is simply an act of turning our minds and our hearts to the sacred. And prayer is not unique to one particular religion.

A recent increased interest in the use of NAC therapies has led to the revisitation of spiritual healing practices. Spiritual healing practices include "faith healing," energy healing such as therapeutic touch, "laying on of the hands," distant healing or healing wishes, meditation, prayer, listening, counseling, psychic healing, and paranormal healing (Dossey, 1999; Rankin-Box, 2001). See Table 11-1 for a list of spiritual healing practices.

The relationship between spirituality and spiritual healing practices and health has been an integral part of the nursing profession since its inception. Although the use of spiritual healing practices started during the time of Florence Nightingale and these practices were popular in the nursing care approaches of early nursing schools, only recently, with the resurgence of NAC therapies, have they begun to gain increasing attention in modern nursing and medicine.

The American Nurses Association (ANA), American Holistic Nurses Association (AHNA), and World Health Organization (WHO) all include spiritual well-being in their definitions of health. Tuck, Pullen, and Wallace (2001) state that prayer is a holistic spiritual healing practice because it is based on the belief that we are all part of the natural harmony of energy in the universe. In spiritual healing, the healer operates from an intention to evolve into a higher power or to channel energy (Patterson, 1998).

TABLE 11-1: EXAMPLES OF SPIRITUAL HEALING PRACTICES

- Religious prayers
- Individual prayers
- Intercessory prayers
- Healing prayers
- General meditations
- Prayerful meditations
- Chinese medicine
- Yoga
- Touch therapy
- Healing rituals
- Dream work
- Distance healing
- Imagery
- Pet therapy
- Music
- Energy healing
  - Reiki
  - Gi gong (vital energy)
  - Polarity
  - Pranic therapy
  - Laying on of hands
  - Therapeutic Touch

Prayer and Faith Healing

Of all the spiritual healing practices, prayer is the one most commonly used. Prayer is defined as "healing intentions or appeals directed toward a higher being, force, or power" (Ameling, 2000). To pray is to ask for something with earnestness or zeal or to supplicate, beg, or give thanks to an object of worship. Prayer can also be defined as "the act of asking for a favor with earnestness or a solemn petition addressed to an object of worship." It can take place in public or private. Ameling (2000) notes that, although the American public generally believes that prayers can cure, prayer is hardly used in practice.

Prayer is not unique to one religion; it is practiced by most of the world's major religions, including Christianity, Judaism, Islam, Hinduism, and Buddhism. In these various religions, beliefs do not always relate to the same god. Some religions may worship more than one god or another higher power. In addition, some religions are guided, not by the word of God, but by prophets, religious founders, and the traditions of the cultures in which they originated. True prayer with dedication can help to achieve moments of transcendence.

Historically, spirituality and prayers have served as personal and communal sources of liberation, solace, hope, meaning, forgiveness, and healing for many people, but especially for African Americans. Spirituality has shaped and promoted individual, family, and communal relationships and is expressed not only by going to church but also in song, music, dance, drumming, art, literature, and health belief practices. When Africans and African Americans are faced with stressful events, such as illness, they often turn to their faith to help them cope. Religion is also used to cope with social, political, and economic injustices. Spirituality is a prominent component of African-American culture (Bourjolly, 1998; Dash, Jackson, & Rasor, 1997; Mattie, 2000; Newlin, Knafl, & Melkus, 2002). Drumming, dance therapy, holy water, visual imagery and, of course, prayer are among some of the spiritual healing practices used in Africa as part of faith healing (Morrison & Thornton, 1999; Wilkinson, Gcabashe, & Lurie, 1999).

Although the WHO is encouraging a shift toward primary health care for developing countries in Africa, the Middle East, and Asia, the economic situations of the majority of their countries have made primary health care practically impossible. Today, many developing countries still have more traditional and faith healers than Western healers. Furthermore, the mixing of these different cultural and religious practices with modern medicine has led to the formation of a new form of medicoreligious practice called *syncretic faith healing,* or simply faith healing. Faith healing is the spiritual acceptance of truth or reality not certified by reason but by the belief in God, a doctrine, or the teaching of a religion. According to Anderson, Anderson, and Glanze (2002), faith healing is to make whole by an alleged healer through the power to cause a cure or recovery from an illness or injury without the aid of conventional medical treatment. Faith healers are believed to have been given their powers by a supernatural force. Faith healers are not only common in Africa but also in Asia, Mexico, and the Middle East, as well as in the Georgia low (coastal) counties of the United States (Anumolu, Miller, Popoola, Talley, & Rushing, 2004).

Some of the experts who have studied or published works on prayer and healing in medicine and health care are Ameling (2000); Dossey (1999, 2000); Dossey and Dossey (1998); Harris et al. (1999); Taylor (2003); and Taylor and Outlaw (2002). Ameling notes that prayer can be both passive and active and that the most private part of prayer is meditation. She also notes that there are seven traditional categories of prayer: petition, intercession, confession, lamentation, adoration, invocation, and thanksgiving.

Buddhist prayer may incorporate the use of a prayer wheel. The prayer wheel, an apparatus used mainly by Buddhists in Tibet, consists of a wheel to which a written prayer is attached. Each revolution of the wheel counts as an utterance of the prayer.

BENEFITS OF SPIRITUAL HEALING PRACTICES

Religious and spiritual healing practices have been used to manage a wide variety of psychological and physical illnesses (Nagai-Jacobson & Burkhardt, 1996, 2001; Huebscher & Shuler, 2003). They positively affect health, decrease morbidity, improve depression and mortality, and increase social support (Luskin et al., 1998; Luskin, 2000). According to Dossey (1993, 1999, 2000), Egan and Arnold (2003), and Jonas and Crawford (2003), spiritual activities have been reported to have the following health and healing benefits:

* grief and bereavement management
* improved quality of life
* decreased abnormal mental behaviors
* reduced drug abuse
* enhanced coping.

In nursing, spiritual healing is considered a part of the holistic approach. In holistic nursing, healing focuses on a person's whole body, mind, and spirit. According to Tuck, Pullen, and Wallace (2001), spiritual healing practices provide comfort and peace, promote wholeness, and enhance coping. In order for nurses to be able to provide spiritual care to clients, nurses must know and appreciate spiritual interventions. Table 11-2 lists nursing interventions that might be acceptable to clients.

RELATED PROFESSIONAL ISSUES

Spirituality is a part of every person's life. According to Walton (1999), spirituality and prayer can provide inner strength, comfort, peace, wellness, and wholeness and can enhance coping for individuals recovering from illness and injury. Whether or not people attend a house of religious practice or subscribe to a doctrine (Huebscher & Shuler, 2004), they can provide spiritual care to others. One need not be a priest, minister, mystic leader, Jewish leader, Muslim leader, reverend, father, or any other religious leader to be able to administer or recommend spirituality to a client.

TABLE 11-2: HOW NURSES CAN PROVIDE SPIRITUAL CARE IN PRACTICE

- Being sensitive to and understanding of other's religious beliefs
- Showing respect for other's spiritual beliefs
- Having the right intention for prayers
- Being open-minded about faith healing, the power of prayer, and other spiritual practices
- Inviting family members to be a part of spiritual care
- Collaborating with clients about providing spiritual care
- Praying with or for clients as needed
- Creating time for clients to visit the hospital chapel
- Encouraging quiet, solitary walks to commune with nature
- Incorporating intercessory prayers (praying for others) as deemed necessary
- Encouraging personal prayers
- Recommending or reminding clients to pray
- Referring to and recommending appropriate religious leaders
- Providing a private place or space for prayer
- Soliciting the help of others in the institution or community
- Encouraging affiliation in a religious community or organization
- Listening to clients who are relating their illness to some spiritual being or power
- Offering spiritual counseling
- Avoiding imposing self-values or beliefs on a client
- Acknowledging the client's concerns for needing spiritual guidance
- Collaborating with religious clergy
- Using touch and silence appropriately in times of spiritual need

Created by Popoola & Clinton, 2004.

Certification is not needed to provide basic spiritual interventions. However, before using any spiritual healing practice or activity as an intervention to promote client healing, a nurse must be comfortable with his or her own spiritual well-being (Tuck, Wallace, & Pullen, 2001). Although certification is not needed to provide certain spiritual care and advice, ethically and legally, a nurse should collaborate with the client or seek the client's permission prior to implementing such practice. Anyone interested in offering spiritual healing as a private practice should seek proper education or experience with a spiritual leader. Nurses are also encouraged to consult with their state licensing board, before setting up a spiritual healing practice.

Although stories and evidence of miraculous healing and cures exist in secular and religious books and in other media, spiritual practices are complementary healing therapies. Caution should be taken before substituting spiritual healing practices for modern medicine. Perhaps the recent development and growth of parish nursing will help nurses to better appreciate spiritual healing in health management. Tuck, Wallace, and Pullen (2001) note that, as parish nurses become an integral part of faith communities, they can also form affiliations with hospitals and create a health care structure that always incorporates spiritual care into practice. In conclusion, there will always be a place for both faith healing and biomedical approaches in holistic healing, especially since science does not fully comprehend life, illness, and death. Until modern science and technology are able to unlock the epistemology (the study of knowledge) and ontology (the study of the nature of existence or being) behind all illnesses, faith healing, life, death, prayers, and spiritual healing, this NAC therapy will continue to be popular.

CONCLUSION

Spiritual healing practice can be found in every culture and it has been in existence since the beginning of civilization. It is sometimes referred to as faith, energy, mystical, shamanic, imaginative, and native healers. However, it should be noted that spiritual healing practice and religions are not one and the same. Prayer, for example, the most commonly use spiritual healing practice, is also common to many religions. However, different religions pray differently and do not always pray to the same God or use prayer as a spiritual healing practice. Faith healing is another type of spiritual healing practice that is also gaining wide recognition as a CAM or NAC therapy.

ONLINE RESOURCES FOR SPIRITUAL HEALING

Empowering Caregivers-Healing
    http://www.care-givers.com

Heart of Healing
    http://www.heartofhealing.net

International Reiki Federation
    http://www.reiki-federation.co.uk/healing.asp

Spiritual Healing
    http://www.dmoz.org/Health/Alternative/
    Energy_Healing

The Transcendent Meditation Program
    http://www.tm.org

EXAM QUESTIONS

CHAPTER 11
Questions 79–85

Note: Choose the one option that BEST answers each question.

79. Shamanism is sometimes associated with

    a. aromatherapy.

    b. aquatic or hydrotherapy.

    c. spiritual healing practice.

    d. guided imagery.

80. One example of a spiritual healing practice is

    a. speaking in tongues.

    b. energy healing.

    c. homeopathy.

    d. shiatsu.

81. The most popular type of spiritual healing is known as

    a. meditation.

    b. shiatsu.

    c. prayer.

    d. shamanism.

82. As a spiritual healing practice, prayer is defined as

    a. spiritual tradition that addresses key elements, such as marriage, rites of passage, and death and dying.

    b. a healing intention or appeal directed toward a higher being, force, or power.

    c. the use of supernatural and mystical powers directed toward a higher being, force, or power.

    d. all of the above.

83. Prayer is practiced by most of the major world religions, including

    a. shamanism.

    b. higher being.

    c. higher power.

    d. Hinduism.

84. Nurses can ethically and legally provide spiritual care in their practice by

    a. insisting that all clients pray before surgery.

    b. following the doctors order for praying.

    c. avoiding imposing spiritual values on clients.

    d. being closed-minded when clients talk about their beliefs.

85. Before setting up a private spiritual healing center, the nurse must check with the

    a. Catholic church.

    b. Board for Parrish Nursing.

    c. state board of nursing.

    d. law board.

CHAPTER 12

RELAXATION THERAPIES: EXERCISE AND HUMOR

CHAPTER OBJECTIVE

Upon completion of this chapter, the leaner will be able to discuss the practice of relaxation therapy and its uses as a holistic alternative and complementary therapy.

LEARNING OBJECTIVES

After studying this chapter, the learner will be able to:

1. Define stress and relaxation.
2. Describe the characteristics of relaxation therapy.
3. Differentiate between the different types of relaxation therapy.
4. List the benefits of relaxation therapy as a holistic alternative and complementary therapy.
5. Identify at least ten different types of relaxation therapy used in stress reduction.
6. Discuss the nursing responsibilities and implications associated with the use of relaxation therapy.

INTRODUCTION

It has been said that laugher is good medicine. However, when most people are in a tense situation, their first response is to get away from the stressful place. Examples of defense mechanisms and stress-reduction strategies used by people when they feel sick, stressed, or worried include taking walks, going for runs, kicking a ball, going to the gym, or simply taking deep breaths. In addition, when one person observes another being sad or tense, that person often tries to cheer the other up with humor or engage him or her in a relaxation activity, such as squeezing a ball. All of these activities are effective therapeutic stress-reducing exercises that help people cope with life's stressors. Unlike binge eating and some other commonly used coping methods, relaxation exercises are safe approaches to the management of stress without adverse effects.

One of the key benefits of every natural, alternative, and complementary (NAC) therapy is stress reduction. "Stress" has become a buzzword in homes and health care environments and many have written about the dangers of stress to health. Stress not only produces stress-related illnesses but is also one of the most common causes of other physical and psychological illnesses in society today. Edwards and Burnard (2003) conducted a systematic review of stress and stress-management interventions, specifically for mental health nurses, and found over 170 papers on the issue. Their review concluded that a great deal of information is currently known about the causes or sources of stress at work, but missing from the literature are the outcomes of interventions for stress reduction (Edwards & Burnard, 2003).

Although thousands of pharmacological agents are available for managing stress, promoting relaxation, and inducing sleep, various

123

nonpharmacological interventions and NAC therapies also exist. NAC therapies commonly used for relaxation include music, meditation, yoga, and herbs (Dossey, 1999). The purpose of this chapter is to briefly discuss three specific types of relaxation therapy: laughter, humor, and exercise therapy.

STRESS

Stress is a real phenomenon. An effect of overactivity of the sympathetic nervous system, stress can produce physical, psychological, social, economic, political, and spiritual imbalance. The wide-ranging effects of stress make it a holistic health issue. The issues of stress, burnout, and stress-related illness have existed in health care since the beginning of nursing and medical practice, and practitioners recognize that stress can cause or contribute to a multitude of illnesses. Stress has been linked to or found to produce such stress-related physical illnesses as hypertension, anxiety disorders, obesity, and headaches. It is also a major cause of psychological illness and spiritual imbalance.

Some examples of causes and results of stress are listed here.

- Physical stress: Heart attack, angina, physical illnesses, open wounds, peptic ulcers, motor vehicle and other accidents
- Psychological stress: Emotional imbalance, panic attacks, depression, psychosis, eating disorders
- Social stress: Group crises, dysfunctional families, family role crises, sociopathy, homelessness
- Economic stress: Inability to pay bills, loss of job or house, bankruptcy, budget crises
- Political stress: Job politics, elections, management, power, arrogant bosses, ineffective employees, political statements, riots, wars
- Spiritual stress: Religious conflict, religious isolation

NAC therapies such as music therapy, herbal therapy, art, dance, exercise, relaxation exercises, humor, and laughter are among the relaxation activities that are commonly used to cope with stress and life stressors. Many health caregivers and the public have also come to realize that hidden away in our bodies, minds, and spirits is the potential for healing. Relaxation activities such as meditation, aquatic therapy, and yoga are commonly used to tap into the body's self-healing potential. Studies on the efficacy of various NAC therapies in the management of stress have been done by many researchers (Coffey, 1999; Dallender, Nolan, Soares, & Thomsen, 1999; Edwards & Burnard, 2003; Richards, Nagel, Markie, Elwell, & Barone, 2003).

DESCRIPTION AND BENEFITS OF RELAXATION THERAPY

"Relaxation" has been defined as the act or the state of being made to be less rigid or tense. It also refers to the absence of physiological or psychological tension and the period when muscles relax between contractions. Many therapeutic interventions can be used to reduce tension and promote a relaxed state. Some such interventions are the use of relaxation activities or exercises. Relaxation therapy and exercises have been used in numerous health care settings to achieve and promote sleep, reduce anxiety, and treat illnesses. They are also commonly used in stressful professions, such as nursing education (Frank, Stephens, & Lee, 1998; Lee, Kawakubo, & Kawamura, 2003; Ulloth, 2002). Relaxation therapy can also be used to promote therapeutic relationships between clients and their family members. Table 12-1 presents some additional benefits of relaxation therapy.

TABLE 12-1: BENEFITS OF RELAXATION THERAPY

- Slows breathing
- Reduces blood pressure
- Relaxes muscles
- Reduces anxiety
- Eliminates stressful thoughts
- Helps clear thinking
- Reduces stress headaches
- Improves focus and concentration
- Assists with elimination of lactic acid and other waste products
- Enhances the immune system
- Reduces pain
- Can be used as an icebreaker
- Can be used in grief management and for hopelessness
- Develops rapport

Tension can lead to emotional, physical, psychological, spiritual, and economic imbalance that can lead to disease. Relaxation exercises are commonly used interventions for anxious patients. This type of therapy has many forms. Most relaxation exercises include breathing exercises. Relaxation activities can bring balance and peace back to the body to facilitate healing of the body, mind, and spirit. Finally, relaxation therapy can create a state of wholeness, and it is the most cost-effective way to promote holistic self-healing.

Types of Relaxation Therapy

Laughter

Three types of relaxation therapy commonly used to promote a relaxed state of mind and body are laughter, humor, and exercise therapy.

Yes, laughter is good medicine. According to Plaskin (2002), research shows that laughter is a holistic tool that is both physically and emotionally therapeutic. It can strengthen the body and invigorate the spirit. Laughter is used to express amusement and can also be used for stress management. Laughter has a potential healing and preventive effect on health and on stress. It can relax muscles, reduce pain, relieve stress, optimize immune function, lower blood pressure, improve circulation, and defuse anger. Humor and laughter have long been used to cope with illness and stress. In fact, the practice dates back to biblical days and the Christian belief that a cheerful heart does good like a medicine, but a broken spirit makes one sick.

Humor

Humor is a state of mind or mood that is used to facilitate how a person perceives, appreciates, and expresses what is funny, amusing, or ludicrous in order to establish relationships, release tension, release anger, facilitate learning, and cope with pain (Rankin-Box, 2001). Writing, speaking, or acting in a comical or amusing way is often considered humorous. According to Buxman (2000), a recognized humorist, humans are all faced with some degree of stress in today's fast-paced life environment, where deadlines, budgets, arrogant bosses, stubborn customers, obstinate teenagers, and bad hair days often determine our states of mind and body. Buxman (2000) notes that whatever the source of stress, the results can be costly if not handled carefully. She recommends the use of laughter and humor as an antidote to life's stressors. As a nurse, Buxman and other health care professionals have been able to combine their skills as storytellers to become humorists who are now training others nationally on how to use humor as a therapeutic exercise for stress management.

Humor and laughter are not necessarily mutually exclusive. Humor can occur without laughter and vice versa. However, laughter is often seen as a physical expression of humor, happiness, jokes, puns, comics, situational comedy, and political satire (Olsson, Backe,

Sorensen, & Kock, 2002). Today, humor is used by all forms of media to promote laughter which, in turn, promotes physical, mental, and spiritual harmony and relaxation.

Exercise Therapy

Exercise therapy is the use of various exercises for the purpose of training or improvement of health. Exercise therapy can range from a simple, relaxing walk in the park to a rigorous training or practice session for fitness and weight loss. Although generally recommended for weight loss, exercise is also frequently recommended for disease management. As discussed here, *exercise therapy* refers to exercises solely intended and carefully selected and tailored to achieve relaxation (Frank, Stephens, & Lee, 1998).

Through exercise therapy, the body can be brought to a state of physical and mental exertion or exhaustion, which can then promote relaxation. Examples of stress-reducing exercise therapies include walking, dancing, swimming, noncompetitive sports, yoga, and pilates. In addition to promoting relaxation and reducing stress, exercise therapy has been proven to be beneficial in

* lowering cholesterol
* lowering blood pressure
* improving sleep
* boosting confidence
* improving immune system function
* protecting the body against injury and disease
* increasing bone density
* improving posture
* increasing oxygen to the bones and muscles.

Every Day Relaxation Activities Used in Stress Reduction

Many different relaxation activities or techniques are used for the management of stress and stress-related illnesses. According to Huebscher and Shuler (2003) and Dossey, Keegan, and Guzzetta (2000), relaxation therapy can be used to manage hypertension, anger,

defensiveness, and stroke. Some strategies include biofeedback, breathing exercise, hypnosis, meditation, music, prayer, creative writing, arts, painting, sculpture, positive social support, support groups, pet therapy, and anger management. The following is a detailed list of the various NAC therapies that can be used to reduce and manage stress. Some have previously been discussed in this course and others are simple, everyday approaches that can be used for stress reduction.

* Aromatherapy: candles, aromas
* Aquatic therapy or hydrotherapy: bubble baths, swimming
* Massage and reflexology: foot or body massage
* Exercise therapy: walking, biking, running, skiing, swimming, kayaking, playing ball or other outdoor games, going to the gym
* Spiritual practices: praying, going to church or a religious center
* Humor: creating humor, reading humorous books, collecting humorous writings and cds
* Laughter: laughing at mistakes, knowing your temperament, chuckling, smiling
* Self-love: reading, understanding one's self-disposition
* Music therapy and poetry: listening to music, playing instruments, singing, writing or reading poetry
* Dance therapy: drumming an instrument
* Yoga and meditation: breathing exercises, stretching
* Guided imagery: imagining whatever is beautiful, comforting, or meaningful
* Time management: not obsessing with time, taking time for self, taking a vacation, getting away and doing fun activities, such as going to a ball game
* Group therapy: joining support groups, creating a social support system
* Art: painting, drawing, sculpting

- Diet: eating right, eating well, eating smart, avoiding self-medication with food
- Group activities: physical or social activities with friends, join groups with common interest – like book, garden, or auto clubs, rediscover face-to-face communication with friends by taking short vacations from social media, texting, emails, etc.

RELATED PROFESSIONAL ISSUES

According to Richards, Nagel, Markie, Elwell and Barone (2003) and Rankin-Box (2001) there is growing evidence from patients, health care professionals, and the public to support the use of relaxation therapies not only for reducing stress but also for managing many illnesses. For example, some humor and laughter research has shown that relaxation exercises boost the immune system (Cheung, Molassiotis, & Chang, 2003; Lower, Bonsack, & Guion, 2003). However, more clinical research is needed to validate the efficacy of these therapeutic modalities.

With few exceptions, exercise therapies carry virtually no risk. However, Rankin-Box (2001) notes that humor is not always effective and might not be appropriate in certain situations. For example, humor and laughter would be totally inappropriate in the acute phase of myocardial infarction but would be appropriate during the rehabilitation or recovery phase of the illness for any age-group. Nurses who intend to use humor and laughter as interventions are encouraged to determine if, and when, humor is appropriate by assessing the timing, the potential receptiveness, the content of the humor, the relationship between the client and the humorist, and the client's belief system.

Humor, laughter, and exercise therapy can be self-administered. In fact, these therapies can be used by anyone and are generally free. Nurses can educate their clients on the various ways to use relaxation therapy. Jokes, puppets, humorous books, movies or cds, games, or funny faces can be used by parents to help relax crying children or to distract them during the performance of a painful procedure. These therapies can also be used to establish rapport and facilitate communication in depressed or critically ill individuals (Dossey, 1998). Relaxation exercises are safe approaches to the management of stress without the adverse effects associated with other coping behaviors, such as drug use and overeating (Frank, Stephens, & Lee, 1998).

CONCLUSION

In conclusion, humor, laughter, and exercise are everyday activities and holistic therapies that can be used as relaxation therapy. Examples of the use of these therapies include dancing, going to a ball game, changing the environment, and properly managing time. Some holistic therapies that can be used to reduce stress include massage, yoga, art, meditation, and aquatic therapy. Nurses can educate clients about the benefits of these relaxation therapies and activities in the management of chronic and stressful illnesses.

ONLINE RESOURCES FOR RELAXATION THERAPIES

Empowering Caregivers-Healing
    http://www.care-givers.com

Holisticonline-Humor
    http://www.holistic-online.com

Laughter Remedy
    http://www.laughterremedy.com

Stress Doctor
    http://www.stressdoc.com

EXAM QUESTIONS

CHAPTER 12
Questions 86–92

Note: Choose the one option that BEST answers each question.

86. Stress is the effect of overactivity of the

    a. parasympathetic nervous system.
    b. sympathetic nervous system.
    c. somatic nervous system.
    d. autonomic nervous system.

87. An example of a relaxation exercise is

    a. running a 10K race.
    b. playing competitive sports.
    c. breathing exercises.
    d. acupuncture.

88. The NAC therapy that is most cost-effective because it is typically free is

    a. relaxation therapy.
    b. massage.
    c. aromatherapy.
    d. vacationing.

89. As types of relaxation therapy, humor and laughter are erroneously considered to be

    a. the only effective types of relaxation therapy.
    b. relaxation therapies that originated from Egypt.
    c. tools for weight management.
    d. mutually exclusive.

90. An exercise therapy that is effective for relaxation is

    a. boxing.
    b. pilates.
    c. lifting weights.
    d. competitive sports.

91. An everyday approach that can be used by anyone for stress reduction is

    a. medication.
    b. shark cartilage therapy.
    c. chelating therapy.
    d. meditation.

92. Some research has shown that humor and laughter can boost the

    a. nervous system.
    b. circulatory system.
    c. immune system.
    d. digestive system.

CHAPTER 13

NUTRITION THERAPY

CHAPTER OBJECTIVE

Upon completion of this chapter, the learner will be able to discuss the history and practice of nutrition therapy and its uses as a holistic alternative and complementary therapy.

LEARNING OBJECTIVES

After studying this chapter, the learner will be able to:

1. Describe the history of nutrition therapy.
2. Recognize the impact of obesity on nutrition therapy.
3. Describe three commonly used weight-loss programs.
4. List ten different types of diet programs.
5. Describe the benefits of a balanced, holistic diet.
6. Discuss key strategies in maintaining a balanced holistic diet.
7. Cite practical applications of nutrition therapy as a holistic alternative and complementary therapy.

INTRODUCTION

Weight-loss advertisements that promise anything and everything are pervasive throughout the media today and fuel a billion dollar industry. It doesn't matter what the product is, the majority of them promise quick and easy weight loss without diet or exercise. If it sounds too good to be true, then it probably is.

Some of these products could even cause health problems. "Don't be hooked by promises, testimonials, or supposed endorsements from reporters; all you'll lose is money" (Federal Trade Commission, 2012).

The Better Business Bureau (BBB) Code of Advertising states that "advertisers should be prepared to substantiate any claims before publication, and also states that claims about performance, efficacy, and results should be based on recent and competent scientific data" (Better Business Bureau, 2013).

In a 2014 article, published in The Journal of the American Medical Association (JAMA), more than one-third of U.S. adults and 17% of youth are obese, although statistics remained unchanged between the years 2003 and 2010 (last data) (Ogdin, Carroll, Kit, & Flegal, 2014). Obesity increases the risk and prevalence of other health problems, such as diabetes, cardiovascular disease, renal disease, cancer, anxiety, and depression. Obesity is also closely linked to stress (Kogut, 2001). Being overweight or obese is not a problem of just the wealthier countries anymore. According to the World Health Organization (WHO, 2014c), obesity has reached epidemic proportions globally, accounting for an annual death rate of at least 2.8 million people.

The effects of obesity are not only physiological but can also be economical, social, psychological, and political. For example, an obese person may not be selected for a certain job due to his or her appearance.

Obesity is a holistic problem that needs a holistic solution. Nutrition therapy involves revisiting our roots to see how to maintain a healthy, nutritious diet of proteins, fats, carbohydrates, vitamins, minerals, fibers, and water in balance. Some of the confusion about nutrition therapy is that we are constantly bombarded with new information about what to eat and what not to eat. Therefore, deciding what to eat has become a "daunting feat" that can be overwhelming (Bright, 2002). When it comes to dieting, staying healthy, and losing weight, the keys are simple: proper nutrition, exercise, lifestyle changes, and behavior modification. A simple formula is to think about how many calories one puts into one's body versus how many calories one burns.

Nutrition therapy is a commonly used natural, alternative, and complementary (NAC) therapy. It is also a part of other NAC therapies, such as naturopathy, herbal therapy, yoga, Chinese medicine, African folk healing, and homeopathy. The purpose of this chapter is to discuss how nutrition therapy can be used as a holistic alternative and complementary therapy. The chapter does not address food groups, present sample menu plans, or list the role of every nutrient in the body. Instead, it addresses key points of nutrition therapy and presents a holistic approach to a balanced diet. Key strategies for achieving balanced, holistic nutrition via self-transformation and behavior (mind) metamorphoses are presented.

HISTORY AND DESCRIPTION

Nutrition is the science of food and its relationship to living beings. To attempt to present the history of nutrition therapy is to attempt to present the history of civilization. Each culture has its own unique way of preparing, eating, and preserving food. People use food not only for physical needs but also for spiritual, economic, social, and psychosocial reasons. Like herbs, the FDA classifies nutrition therapy as diet supplements.

From the Prehistoric Age to the Stone Age, our ancestors survived primarily on diets consisting of natural resources, such as plants. Their diets depended on their hunting, fishing, planting, and food-gathering skills. Food additives and food processing technologies were not available to them, and they did not have to count calories or watch what they ate. The food available to prehistoric man was based on geographical location and the natural resources available. For example, cultures that lived close to wildlife fed on animals, whereas cultures that lived close to water fed on fish. This is one reason for varying food preferences among different cultures. According to Lutz and Przytulski (2001), the traditional diet of the Eskimos, for example, consisted mostly of fish, whereas the diets of other Native American tribes consisted mostly of fruits.

Food is critical to our existence. It provides us with the nutrients necessary for body functioning, survival, and energy. However, food shapes us not only physically but also psychologically. According Geary (2000), more than 50% of all overweight people not only suffer from physical and psychological problems with food, but they use food to cope with other problems, such as depression, anger, and stress.

Nutrition therapy is becoming increasingly popular as a stand-alone NAC therapy; however, it can also be used as part of other NAC therapies, such as naturopathy, herbal therapy, yoga, ayurveda, Chinese medicine, and homeopathy (Geary, 2000). Nutrition therapy is also a holistic healing aspect of many folk healing practices (Huebscher & Shuler, 2003; Cataldo, DeBruyne, & Whitney, 2003).

Being overweight or obese increases the risk of many diseases and health conditions, such as hypertension, high cholesterol and triglycerides, type 2 diabetes, coronary heart disease, stroke, gallbladder disease, osteoarthritis, sleep apnea, respiratory problems, and some types of cancer (CDC, 2014b). Diet treatments work only on a short-term basis rather than on the holistic healing model. According to Miller (2001), because of the obesity epidemic, traditional diet and exercise are no longer effective; rather, behavior and maintenance plans should be key strategies in the management of weight problems. Treatment that simply focuses on diet, exercise, and behavior modification cannot solve this epidemic problem. A paradigmatic shift in thinking is required from the mechanistic way of viewing life, illness, stress, and treatment to a holistic view that promotes healing rather than temporary curing. Nutrition therapy and dieting must be approached as a holistic healing modality for treatment to be successful and to avoid the yo-yo effects of dieting. Florence Nightingale (1859) was the first nurse to introduce the use of proper nutrition to promote self-healing and prevent and manage disease.

KEY POINTS IN NUTRITION THERAPY

Calories

Calories are important in nutrition therapy but should not become an obsession. Calorie count has become a buzz phrase with diets and in the management of such disease as diabetes and obesity. Counting calories, however, does not need to be rigorous and obsessive. According to Bright (2002) and Cataldo, DeBruyne, and Whitney (2003), because many foods are processed or genetically modified (GMO), many diseases or nutritional deficiencies now exist due to the production of certain toxins. Eating five slices of cake, for example, simply because it is made with little, or no calories gives a person a false or temporary fix for a problem that requires a long-term solution. Obesity is a chronic problem and, like other chronic illnesses, it simply reappears the moment people stop counting points or calories (Eliopoulos, 2004). Eating naturally and sensibly is a more effective and holistic solution.

A calorie is defined by Webster (1979) as a unit of heat or the unit expressing heat or energy potential of food when digested. To translate calories into weight gain and loss is simply to think in terms of heat loss or gain. To understand calories, it can help to think in terms of the calories that certain foods contain. For example:

- Protein produces 4 kilocalories per 1 g.
- Carbohydrates produce 4 kilocalories per 1 g.
- Fat produces 9 kilocalories per 1 g.
- Alcohol produces 7 kilocalories per 1 g.
- Water, fiber, vitamins, and minerals do not produce any kilocalories.

Fat is critical for daily mental and metabolic processes; thus, it must be included in our meals. However, because it produces more calories than protein and carbohydrates, fat intake should be limited. Because fiber, vitamins, and minerals can be gained from eating naturally acquired, prepared and nonprocessed fats, carbohydrates, and proteins, experts tell us that we do not have to think about getting the right vitamins, minerals, and fiber if we eat properly and naturally. However, when people focus on calories and points and look for ways to cheat by eating processed and refined foods with low caloric and artificial ingredients, they run the risk of not just temporarily losing weight but also losing vitamins, minerals, and fiber that are needed for biological functioning. For example, many vitamins and minerals are co-enzymes necessary for the metabolism of fat, carbohydrates, and protein. Although water, fiber, vitamins, and minerals are considered empty calories, their roles in metabolism and cell functioning should not be underestimated or taken lightly. Technically, calories from fat and carbohydrates are needed for energy and protein is needed for repairing injured tissue. When the body does not receive proper nutrition, these roles can be reversed and create a state of metabolic imbalance.

Cultural and Personal Food Preferences

No two people like to eat all the same foods. Food preferences vary, especially from culture to culture. Food tastes are like imprints or permanent markers. Also, people commonly use food from their native countries as a socialization tool and common bond and attempts to create a diet that will work for everyone is not only impossible but also impractical. Nutrition therapy must therefore address and explore food preferences within a cultural context and food recommendations must be modified appropriately.

Since the days of our ancestors, nutritional habits have been influenced not only by geographical location and the availability of resources but by agriculture, adaptation, economics, famine, food storage issues, cultural and religious views, and the relationship between diet and health in that culture (Lutz & Przytulski, 2001). Nutritional beliefs are attached to certain foods by different cultures. The process of preparing, combining, and serving the basic food groups also varies from culture to culture. It is not unusual now for people to substitute drinking water with soft drinks or other high-caloric beverages, without decreasing caloric intake from another dietary source. Food portions are often super-sized and high in sugars and fats, with easy accessibility and overwhelming abundance.

Lutz and Przytulski (2001) note that food items vary widely from culture to culture and are influenced by economical, religious, health, and geographical constraints. Cultural influences and preferences should be considered in the use of nutrition therapy for healing or disease management. Understanding the various types of food that have symbolic and health meanings to cultures is also important. The Chinese philosophy of yin and yang is referred to by some as Zen macrobiotics (Pulver, 1998). Also, coconut is used by many cultures for nutritional and medicinal purposes (Huebscher & Shuler, 2003). The coconut as a holistic and functional fruit will be discussed later in this chapter.

POPULAR DIETS COMMONLY USED FOR WEIGHT LOSS

Because of the availability today of so many types of diets, deciding which plan is best for a person can be overwhelming. When it comes to the management of diseases, specifically cancer and diabetes, Kogut (2001) and Dyson (2002) not only discuss the role of nutrition therapy in the management of these conditions but provide the many types of diets that are commonly used. Many fad diets, such as the grapefruit diet, have come and gone. It should be noted that in almost all diet programs, exercise and regular physical activity should be recommended (Miller, 2001). According to Miller (2001), exercise is the only variable that consistently shows effectiveness in physiological, medical, psychological, and behavioral outcomes of obesity. Three specific popular diet programs are described in this section, and Table 13-1 presents other diet programs commonly used today.

TABLE 13-1: DIET PROGRAMS

- Zone Diet
- Australian Zone Diet
- Hot and Cold Zone Diet
- Low-carb diet
- Protein diet
- High-protein diet
- South Beach Diet
- Paleo diet
- Gerson therapy
- Macrobiotic diet
- Blood-type diet
- Traditional diet
- Asian diet
- Latin American diet
- Vegetarian diet
- Vegan diet
- Gluten-free diet

- Low-fat diet
- Mediterranean diet
- Millennium Diet
- Weight Watchers
- Mayo Clinic Diet
- Cyber Diet
- Jenny Craig
- Juice therapy
- Pritikin Diet
- Whole food diet
- Diamond Diet
- Elimination diet
- Fasting
- Slim Fast Diet
- Nutrisystem Diet
- Weigh Down Diet

The **Atkins diet** is a popular low-carbohydrate, high-protein diet. It is based on the principles of restriction of processed and refined carbohydrates and limited consumption of sugar, breads, pasta, and starchy vegetables. In the Atkins diet, there is an initial two-week period during which ketosis is induced.

The **Mediterranean diet** is one diet that is frequently noted to be successful because it is based on eating traditional, nonprocessed foods that are limited in sugar. Fruits, rather than desserts containing refined sugar, are commonly recommended. Food recommendations include locally grown fresh fruits and vegetables, nuts, grains, and seeds. Olive oil is a key ingredient in all cooking on this diet. It is considered a very healthy diet that improves health and longevity. The majority of the foods are plant-based, with limited animal food sources. Instead of meat, fish is used for protein. The Mediterranean diet contains abundant micronutrients that are commonly lost in processed or fertilized foods.

Vegetarian and Vegan diets are often low in saturated fats and high in fiber, vitamins, and phytochemicals. These diets are used not only for personal reasons but also for religious and health reasons. Not all vegetarian diets lack animal products. Vegetarian diets may include dairy products and eggs. Vegan diets are strictly plant-based.

BENEFITS OF PROPER NUTRITION

Since obesity and stress are the roots of many illnesses today, the benefit of proper nutrition is not only to maintain an ideal body weight but to prevent and manage illness. For example, vitamin C and zinc can be used in the management and prevention of respiratory infections, such as colds, sore throats, and sinusitis as well as in the promotion of wound healing (Huebscher & Shuler, 2003). Generally, the benefits of proper nutrition are to build the body's reserves, help to build the immune system to prevent illness, and help the body function optimally. Proper nutrition can also help to prevent obesity and many of its debilitating complications, such as diabetes, hypertension, asthma, and back pain, to mention just a few.

KEY STRATEGIES IN BALANCED HOLISTIC NUTRITION

When faced with unpleasant emotions or disappointments or overcome by stress, anxiety, or depression, the body has a natural instinct to respond. For many people, this response involves eating. It is important to understand the role of stress in dieting, particularly because unresolved stress can induce physiologic changes. For example, in response to stress, the body releases hormones that stimulate appetite and cravings, prompting the intake of huge quantities of fattening and high-carbohydrate foods. Because of the physiologic interaction between stress and eating, it is important to use NAC therapies that reduce stress and promote relaxation to avoid abuse of food.

Basics of Balanced Holistic Nutrition

The goal of balanced holistic nutrition is to eat smart and naturally. This involves the following recommendations:

- Choose vibrantly colored fruits and vegetables as they are rich in phytochemicals, antioxidants, flavonoids, carotenoids, anthocyanins, lycopene and essential vitamins, minerals and fiber.
- Eat a balanced diet to meet the recommended daily allowance of vitamins, minerals, and fiber.

- Avoid high fructose, sugary beverages with empty calories; drink water.
- Avoid eating when feeling stressed, upset, sad, disappointed, or happy – emotional eating
- Omit or decrease trans fat snacks. Instead eat healthy snacks such as protein-containing snacks that are filling, and fresh fruits and vegetables.
- Eat consistently and sensibly.
- Eat natural foods that have not been processed, altered, or refined.
- Eat smaller portions. Eat slowly. Eat only when hungry. Stop when full. Listen to your body.
- Avoid yo-yo dieting.
- Reduce intake of saturated fats, trans fatty acids (trans fats), hydrogenated and partially hydrogenated oils, Substitute "good" fats such as those found in nuts, olives, and avocados.
* Replace sauces, high in fats, sugars, sodium and chemicals, with vinegars, mustards, and lemon juice. Add fresh herbs and spices for flavor.
- Know your body mass index.
- Start an exercise program.
- Change eating habits and lifestyle.
- Set long-term goals and stay focused on them. Remember that no quick fix or cure exists for obesity.

Self-Transformation and Mind (Behavioral) Metamorphoses

Change is an inevitable part of life, and it is necessary before weight loss can begin. For example, people must learn to handle stress. Self-determination and goals are critical. Nutrition therapy and diet modification are about mind over matter (body), and a balanced holistic life and diet are necessary. No medicine, no fad diet, and no nurse, dietician, or doctor can make this happen for a person. Some fad diets have side effects, lack balanced nutrition, and discourage self-control; many focus on curing, which provides only a temporary solution. People on these diets commonly gain back all of the weight they have lost, and sometimes more, when discontinuing the diet.

For nutrition therapy to be effective and long lasting, people must be willing to control and manage what they eat and must be willing to change their philosophy of life. Nutrition therapy is about living holistically and taking care of oneself – a holistic self-care approach. The bottom line is that to lose 1 pound, a person must be willing and able to decrease food intake by 3,500 calories – equivalent to 1 pound – or increase activity or caloric loss by the same amount. Losing weight can take days, weeks, or months. However, it may take just one meal to consume 3,500 calories. A balanced holistic diet focuses on maintaining homeostasis and understanding that food cravings and overeating have emotional components and physiological side effects – overweight and obesity.

RELATED PROFESSIONAL ISSUES

Before discussing nutrition therapy with a client, careful exploration of individual cultural differences are critical. For example, when discussing nutrition therapy with someone from India, it is important to address his or her belief in Ayurveda, a traditional, comprehensive health care system which dates back 5,000 years and places heavy emphasis on nutrition therapy. Nurses and other health care providers who are interested in holistic nutrition management should consult specific books, schools, and internet resources about the government regulations, standards, and specifics regarding certification.

Although there are dieticians and nutritionists who are specifically trained to address nutrition needs of clients, in many cases their views are not holistic. Current teaching approaches are often from a mechanistic worldview where exchange lists and measurement of food intake are still the focuses. The holistic approach to nutrition and diet according to Eliopoulos (2004) considers self-care, healthful food selection, moderate intake, and balance. This holistic approach to dieting and healthy eating empowers clients to use common sense and inner wisdom to balance their food intake while maintaining a balanced lifestyle for the body, mind, and spirit.

CONCLUSION

Food is like fuel for the body. When a person puts the right kind of fuel into his or her body, the body functions properly. However, with the wrong type of food, the body can incur problems or diseases. To maintain balanced holistic nutrition, one must also exercise and make lifestyle changes. Nutrition therapy is both an alternative and complementary therapy in that it can, and should, be used not just for disease management but also for disease prevention.

Nutrition therapy is a part of other CAM and NAC therapies. Regardless of the stressors and illnesses one encounters in life, the use of proper nutrition and other types of CAM (such as herbal therapy, aromatherapy, massage therapy, reflexology, music therapy, touch therapy, yoga, meditation, aquatic therapy, folk healing practices, spiritual healing practices, homeopathy, acupuncture, Chinese medicine, exercise therapy, humor and laughter, relaxation exercises, guided imagery) discussed in this book can always be used to achieve and maintain a sense of balance and homeostasis. Health care providers, especially nurses, can openly teach patients holistic and self-care approaches to healing. Our role as health care providers and as nurses is to begin open, honest, and positive dialogues with our patients and ourselves when it comes to living healthy lifestyles with proper nutrition and holistic balance.

Nutrition therapy from a holistic perspective requires a paradigmatic shift to a nutrition approach that is balanced and requires us to eat smartly, naturally and, most importantly, it requires a self-behavioral metamorphoses.

ONLINE RESOURCES FOR NUTRITION THERAPY

American Dietary Guideline
http://www.healthierus.gov/dietaryguidelines

Diet, Nutrition & Eating Right
http://www.health.gov/DietaryGuidelines

Centers for Disease Control and Prevention (CDC)
http://www.cdc.gov/nutrition

United States Department of Agriculture (USDA) – Food and Nutrition Information Center
http://fnic.nal.usda.gov/dietary-supplements/complementary-and-alternative-medicine

Food and Drug Administration (FDA) – Food
http://www.fda.gov/Food/default.htm

Food and Drug Administration (FDA) – Food Plate
http://www.choosemyplate.gov

Holistic Healing – Holistic Nutrition
http://www.healing.about.com

Institute of Holistic Nutrition
http://www.instituteofholisticnutrition.com

National Center for Complementary and Alternative Medicine (NCCAM)
http://nccam.nih.gov

United States Department of Agriculture (USDA) – Weight Management & Calories
http://www.choosemyplate.gov/weight-management-calories.html

EXAM QUESTIONS

CHAPTER 13
Questions 93–100

Note: Choose the one option that BEST answers each question.

93. Nutrition therapy is also considered a part of

    a. music therapy.

    b. aromatherapy.

    c. herbal therapy.

    d. aquatic therapy.

94. The FDA classifies herbs and nutrition therapy as

    a. drugs.

    b. dietary supplements.

    c. health education.

    d. holistic food.

95. The nursing theorist who first addressed the importance of nutrition therapy and health is

    a. Watson.

    b. Orem.

    c. Nightingale.

    d. Rogers.

96. A unit of food measurement is known as

    a. protein.

    b. macrobiotic.

    c. calorie.

    d. alcohol.

97. The fruit that is referred to as a "functional food" is the

    a. orange.

    b. onion.

    c. coconut.

    d. walnut.

98. The popular diet program that focuses on high intake of protein is

    a. calories diet.

    b. exchange list.

    c. vegetarian diet.

    d. Atkins diet.

99. A balanced holistic diet program should be based on

    a. counting points.

    b. counting calories.

    c. eating limited carbohydrates.

    d. eating smart.

100. A traditional comprehensive health care system that has been practiced in India for more than 5,000 years is

    a. Chinese medicine.

    b. African folk healing.

    c. ayurveda.

    d. meditation.

This concludes the final examination.

Please answer the evaluation questions found on page v of this course book.

GLOSSARY

acupressure: Use of touch of the pressure points and meridians in the management of illness. The points in acupressure correspond to the acupuncture points, but the stimulation in acupressure is achieved not with needles but rather with finger pressure and touching.

acupuncture: Use of needle piercing to regulate or correct the flow of chi (energy) to restore health.

aphorism: A principle expressed in a few words or a brief sentence containing some important truths or a brief statement of a doctrine.

aquatic therapy: The use of water in the treatment of various disorders that may include continuous tub baths, wet sheet packs, or shower sprays. Also see Chapter 6.

axiom: An established rule or principle or a self-evident truth. An aphorism.

ayurveda: A form of holistic alternative medicine that is the traditional or folk system of medicine in India.

biofeedback: Use of an instrument to mirror psychophysiological processes of which an individual is not normally aware and which may be brought under voluntary control.

buoyancy factor: The force of gravity that results in a feeling of weightlessness when immersed in water. A term used to describe one of the properties of water.

calories: A measurement unit of energy or a unit equaling the amount of heat required to raise the temperature of 1 gram of water 1 degree Celsius. Shortened form for kilocalories.

centering: A sense of self-relatedness that can be thought of as a place of inner being or place of quietude within oneself where one can feel truly integrated, unified, and focused.

chakra: One of the body's seven energy centers that serve as the basis for some holistic healing therapies, such as yoga and meditation. They are the openings that allow life energy to flow into and out of the aura.

chanting: The act of singing a song of short, repetitive melody used in liturgical singing characterized by single notes to which as many syllabuses as required are assigned. Examples include a psalm or any monotonous song.

chelating agent: A chemical compound that binds metallic ions into a ring structure, inactivating them, and can be used to remove poisonous metals from the body.

chi: In Chinese medicine, body energy or basic life energy. Also "qi."

coenzyme: A substance that combines with an enzyme to activate it.

daydreaming: An abstract or concrete visionary fantasy, usually spontaneous, that is indulged in while awake to provide inner information.

dermabrasion: The act of rubbing, cupping, pinching, rubbing, and burning to erode or grate off.

dreams: Conscious awareness of images, visions, and thoughts during sleep or daydreaming. Spontaneous imagery that primarily involves the visual mode, may be concrete or abstract, and provides a person with inner phenomena that can be therapeutic.

drum (drumming): A musical instrument of the percussive class, consisting of a hollow body covered at one or both ends with a tightly stretched membrane, or head, which is struck with sticks or a hand to produce sounds.

efficacy: The ability of a drug to achieve the desired effect.

energy: The capacity to do work.

enfleurage: The process of extracting perfumes by exposing inodorous oils or fats to the exhalations from flowers. Used when flower oils are too delicate or fugitive to undergo distillation.

enzyme: Complex protein produced by living cells that acts as a catalyst.

expression: Method used exclusively to extract essential oils from citrus fruits. When the peel is mechanically pressed, droplets of oil and juice are squeezed out and separated.

guided imagery: Visualization. The internal experience of memories, dreams, fantasies, and visions that serves as the bridge for connecting body, mind, and spirit.

herbalists: Folk healers skilled in the use of herbs, roots, and plants to treat common disorders

holism: 1. philosophical theory: the view that a whole system of beliefs must be analyzed rather than simply its individual components
2. theory of health: the theory of the importance of taking all of somebody's physical, mental, and social conditions into account in the treatment of illness

homeopathy: The system of treating disease by administering in minute quantities drugs that, if given in larger doses to a healthy person, would produce symptoms similar to those of the disease.

homeopathists: Are local chemists or pharmacists who mix extracts from roots, teas, or plants for medicinal purposes. This practice cuts across many countries.

hydrotherapy: See "aquatic therapy."

hypnosis: A trancelike state resembling sleep that is artificially induced and characterized by a marked susceptibility to suggestion and considerable loss of willpower and sensation.

hypnotherapy: Use of hypnosis to treat mental and physical diseases.

hypnotic: A drug, sedative, or other agent that produces sleep.

iatrogenic: Any adverse mental and physical condition induced in a patient by effects of treatment and surgery.

maceration: A labor-intensive and costly method of extracting essential oils that involves steeping a plant in a liquid in order to extract soluble constituents. Can be performed with or without heat.

massage therapy: The process of using the hands to apply pressure and motion to the skin and underlying muscle of a client for the purpose of physical and psychological relaxation, improvement of circulation, relief of sore muscles, and other therapeutic purposes.

meditation: The art of meditating (dwelling on something in thought) or the revolving of a subject in the mind. Also, a state of intense awareness achieved by intensely concentrating on a single object until all other thoughts vanish.

meridian: An energy circuit or line of force that runs vertically and flows through the body with concentrated points on the feet, arms, and ears. Meridian lines and zones influence the use of pressure points. Channels or conduits through which chi flows or travels in the body. Used in acupuncture, shiatsu, and many other alternative and complementary therapies.

mineral: An inorganic element or compound necessary for human life.

music therapy: The use of music to enhance, improve, and maintain physical, emotional, economic, political, and spiritual well-being.

naturopathy: A system of therapeutics based on natural foods, light, warmth, massage, fresh air, regular exercise, and the avoidance of medication. Advocates believe that the natural processes of the body can heal disease.

nutrition: The science of food and its relationship to living beings.

poultice: A warm moist preparation placed on an aching or inflamed part of the body to ease pain, improve circulation, or hasten the expression of pus.

prayer: The act of turning the mind and the heart to the sacred, or the act of asking for a favor with earnestness or a solemn petition addressed to an object of worship in public or in private.

prehistoric: Period of time before humans could write.

reflexology: A system of treating certain disorders by massaging the soles of the feet or palms of the hand using principles similar to those of acupuncture.

relaxation: A state of consciousness characterized by a feeling of peace and release of tension, anxiety, and fear or the absence of physical, mental, and emotional tension.

shamanism: A religion practiced by many cultures that is characterized by spiritual healing (herbalism). Shamans are community leaders who operate based on a state of consciousness to fulfill certain social and cultural non-health-related obligations to their communities, such as marriage, rites of passage, death and dying, parenting, and growth.

shiatsu: Literally, "finger pressure." A therapy in which the practitioner uses the thumb or heel of the hand to apply deep pressure along the lines of the meridians. A hands-on therapy that works on the energy pathways to balance and strengthen the body in order to facilitate self-healing and relaxation and provide support for general health and well-being.

solvent extraction: Extraction of aromatic compounds using hydrocarbon solvents. A solvent-extracted scent, or fragrance, always has a slight petroleum smell, which may or may not affect the aroma or therapeutic benefit.

sound: A noise, musical tone, or vocal utterance. The sensation produced in the organ of hearing by certain vibrations, or sound waves, conveyed by the atmosphere, water, or other elastic media.

standardization: Provides a measure of quality control that ensures all batches of a product are consistently uniform.

steep: To soak. A process used in maceration extraction of essential oils.

stress: The effect of overactivity of the sympathetic nervous system.

synthetics: The use of the science of organic chemistry or compounds that mimic living organisms to create essential oils in a laboratory. The process of making essential oils without having to use real ingredients.

Therapeutic Touch: A specific technique of centering intention used while a practitioner moves the hands through a recipient's energy fields for the purpose of assessment and treatment of energy field imbalance. A form of touch therapy.

touch therapy: A broad range of techniques used by a practitioner that involve placing the hands on or near the body to assist a patient toward optimal functioning or healing. Examples include massage therapy, Therapeutic Touch, shiatzu, and reflexology.

vitamin: An organic element or substance necessary for normal growth, metabolism, and development of the body that is important in energy transformation and also acts as a coenzyme in the enzymatic system.

yoga: Literally, "to join together." A system of techniques that enables the joining of the physical, emotional, and spiritual bodies.

yo-yo effect: The repeated loss and gain of body weight.

zones: A term used in reflexology for areas of specific boundary of energy pathways.

REFERENCES

Ai, A.L., Peterson, C., Bolling, S.F., & Koenig, H.G. (2002). Private prayer and optimism in middle-aged and older patients awaiting cardiac surgery. *Gerontologist, 42*(1), 70-81.

Ai, A.L., Peterson, C., Gillespie, B., Bolling, S.F., Jessup, M.G. (2004). Association of Reflexologists. *Delivering excellence in reflexology.* http://www.aor.org.uk

Ai, A., Peterson, C., Gillespie, B., Bolling, S.F., Jessup, M.G., Behling, B.A., et al. (2001). Designing clinical trails on energy healing: Ancient art meets medical science. *Alternative Therapies in Health and Medicine, 7*(4), 83-90.

Ai, A.L., Peterson, C., Tice, T.N., Bolling, S.F., & Koenig, H.G. (2004). Faith-based and secular pathways to hope and optimism: Subconstructs in middle-aged and older cardiac patients. *Journal of Health Psychology, 9*(3), 435-50.

Aworldofaromatherapy.com. (n.d.). *History of Aromatherapy.* http://www.aworldofaroma therapy.com/aromatherapy-origins.htm

Allaire, A.D., Moos, M.K., & Wells, S.R. (2000). Complementary and alternative medicine in pregnancy: A survey of North Carolina certified nurse-midwives. *Obstetrics and Gynecology, 95*(1), 19-23.

Ameling, A. (2000). Prayer: An ancient healing practice becomes new again. *Holistic Nursing Practice, 14*(3), 40-48.

American Botanical Council (ABC). (2013). HerbalGram is the peer-reviewed quarterly journal of the nonprofit American Botanical Council, *Herbal Dietary Supplement Retail Sales Up 5.5% in 2012.* http://cms.herbalgram. org/press/2013/2012_Market_Report.html

American Cancer Society (ACS). (2014a). *Music Therapy.* http://www.cancer.org/treatment/ treatmentsandsideeffects/complementary andalternativemedicine/mindbodyandspirit/ music-therapy

American Cancer Society (ACS). (2014b). *Therapeutic Touch.* http://www.cancer.org/ treatment/treatmentsandsideeffects/comple mentaryandalternativemedicine/manual healingandphysicaltouch/therapeutic-touch

American Holistic Nurses Association. (2000). *AHNA standards of holistic nursing practice: Guidelines for caring and healing.* Gaithersburg, MD: Aspen Publishers.

American Holistic Nurses Association. (2014). *Descriptions of healing modalities.* http:// www.ahna.org/Home/For-Consumers/ Holistic-Modalities

American Institute of Holistic Theology (AIHT). (2014). *Chakras.* http://www.aiht.edu/door ways/chakra_door.asp?adclfr=THCOM

American Institute of Holistic Theology (AIHT). (2014). *Metaphysics.* http://www.aiht.edu/ catalog/metaphysics.asp

American Music Therapy Association (AMTA). (n.d.). *A Career in Music Therapy.* http:// www.musictherapy.org/careers/employ ment/#APPROVED_CURRICULUM

American Massage Therapy Association (AMTA). (2014). *Massage: Becoming a massage therapist.* http://www.amtamassage.org

American Reflexology Certification Board (ARCB). (2014). http://arcb.net/cms

American Yoga Association. (2005a). *General information about yoga.* http://american yogaassociation.org/contents.html

American Yoga Association. (2005b). *How to choose a qualified teacher.* http://www.americanyogaassociation.org/teachers.html

American Yoga Association. (2005c). *Yoga and wellness.* http://www.americanyogaassociation.org/wellness.html

American Yoga Association. (2005d). *Yoga A to Z.* http://www.americanyogaassociation.org/Yoga%20A%20to%20Z.html

Anderson, K.N., Anderson, L.E., & Glanze, W.D. (2002). *Mosby's medical, nursing, & allied health dictionary* (6th ed.). St. Louis: Mosby.

Anumolu, A., Miller, H., Popoola, M., Talley, B., & Rushing, A. (2004). Alternative health care systems. In R. Huebscher and P.A. Shuler, *Natural, alternative, and complementary health care practices* (pp. 715-61). St. Louis: Mosby.

Arnold, J. (1996). The healing power of touch. *New Woman, 26*(7), 82-85.

Astin, J.A., Shapiro, S.L., Eisenberg, D.M., & Forys, K.L. (2003). Mind-body medicine: State of the science, implications for practice. *Journal of the American Board of Family Practice, 16*(2), 131-47.

Ataudo, E.S. (1985). Traditional medicine and biopsychosocial fulfillment in Africa health. *Social Science & Medicine, 21*(12), 1345-47.

Auckett, A. (1989). *Baby massage: Parent-child bonding through touch.* New York: Newmarket Press.

Avis, A. (1999). Aromatherapy in practice. *Nursing Standard, 13*(24), 14-15.

Ballard, C.G., O'Brien, J.T., Reichelt, K., & Perry, E.K. (2002). Aromatherapy as a safe and effective treatment for the management of agitation in severe dementia: The results of a double-blind, placebo-controlled trial with Melissa. *Journal of Clinical Psychiatry, 63*(7), 553-58.

Barrios, J. (1999). Is herbal therapy helpful or hazardous? *Journal of the American Dietetic Association, 99*(5), 530.

Becker, B. & Cole, A. (1997). *Comprehensive aquatic therapy.* London, Butterworth-Heinemann.

Benfield, R.D. (2002). Hydrotherapy in labor. *Journal of Nursing Scholarship, 34*(4), 347-52.

Benfield, R.D., Herman, J., Katz, V.L., Wilson, S.P., & Davis, J.M. (2001). Hydrotherapy in labor. *Journal of Nursing Scholarship, 24*(1), 57-67.

Benkel, D.H., McClure, E.M., Woolard, D., Rullan, J.V., Miller, G.B., Jenkins, S.R., et al. (2000). Outbreak of Legionnaires' disease associated with a display whirlpool spa. *International Journal of Epidemiology, 29*(6), 1092-1098.

Benson, S. (1997). Music as medicine for the terminally ill. *Holistic Health News, 5*(6), 7-8.

Bernatzky, G. (2003). Tune out your back pain. (Interview). *Natural Health, 33*(2), 26-27.

Better Business Bureau (BBB). (2013). *The skinny on weight loss advertising.* http://www.bbb.org/blog/2013/05/the-skinny-on-weight-loss-advertising

BioSpiritual Energy Healing. (n.d.). *Essential oil chemistry of our biospiritual allies.* http://www.biospiritual-energy-healing.com/essential-oil-chemistry.html

Black, P.K. (2000). *Holistic stoma care.* Bailliere-Tindall. Edinburgh, London: Harcourt.

Blanc, P.D., Trupin, L., Earnest, G., Katz, P.P., Yelin, E.H., Eisner, M.D. (2001). Alternative therapies among adults with a reported diagnosis of asthma or rhinosinusitis: Data from a population-based survey. *Chest, 120*(5), 1461-67.

Blumenthal, M. (1998). *The complete German commission E monographs.* Boston: Integrative Medicine Communications.

Blumenthal, M., Goldberg, A., & Brinckmann, J. (2000). *Herbal medicine: Expanded commission E monographs.* Newton, MA: American Botanical Council.

Bonny, H. (1983). Music listening for intensive coronary care units: A pilot project. *Music Therapy, 3*(1), 4.

Bonny, H. & Savary, L. (1973). *Music and your mind: Listening with a new consciousness.* New York: Harper & Row.

Bourjolly, J.N. (1998). Differences in religiousness among black and white women with breast cancer. *Social Work in Health Care, 28*(1), 21-39.

Breiner, M. (1993). Whole body dentistry – excerpt from chapter 2, *A Paradigm Shift.* http://www.altmedangel.com/paradigm.htm

Bright, M.A. (2002). *Holistic health and healing.* Philadelphia: F.A. Davis Company.

Broach, E. & Dattilo, J. (1996). Aquatic therapy: A viable therapeutic recreation intervention. *Therapeutic Recreation Journal, 30*(3), 213-27.

Broach, E., Groff, D., & Dattilo, J. (1997). Effects of an aquatic therapy-swimming program on adults with spinal cord injuries. *Therapeutic Recreation Journal, 31*(3), 160-173.

Brygge, T., Heinig, J.H., Collins, P., Ronborg, S.M., Gehrchen, P.M., Hilden, J., et al. (2002). Zone therapy and asthma. *Ugeskrift for Laeger, 164*(18), 2405-2410.

Buckle, J. (1997). *Clinical Aromatherapy in Nursing.* London: Arnold Publishers.

Buckle, J. (1999). Use of aromatherapy as a complementary treatment for chronic pain. *Alternative Therapies in Health and Medicine, 5*(5), 42-51.

Buckle, J. (2001). The role of aromatherapy in nursing care. *The Nursing Clinics of North America, 36*(1), 57-72.

Bullough, V. & Bullough, B. (1993). Therapeutic touch: Why do nurses believe? *The Skeptical Inquirer, 17*(2) 169-174.

Burns, S. & Burns, J. (2000). Massage therapy. *The Journal of Alternative and Complementary Medicine, 6*(3), 217-18.

Burns, S.J., Harbuz, M.S., Hucklebridge, F., & Bunt, L. (2001). A pilot study into the therapeutic effects of music therapy at a cancer help center. *Alternative Therapies in Health and Medicine, 7*(1), 48-56.

Buxman, K. (2000). Humor in critical care: No joke. *AACN Clinical Issues, 11*(1), 120-27.

Campbell, A. (2000). Acupuncture, touch, and the placebo response. *Complementary Therapies in Medicine, 8*(1), 43-46.

Campbell, D.G. (1997). *The Mozart effect: Tapping the power of music to heal the body, strengthen the mind, and unlock the creative spirit.* New York: Avon Books.

Canter, P.H. (2003). The therapeutic effects of meditation. *BMJ, 326*(7398), 1049-50.

Canyon Ranch. (2013). *Reflexology for better health.* http://www.canyonranch.com/your-health/health-healing/healing-therapies/touch-therapies/reflexology-better-health#fbid=DcChErfLgo7

Carlsson, C. (2002). Acupuncture mechanisms for clinically relevant long-term effects: Reconsideration and a hypothesis. *Acupuncture in Medicine: Journal of the British Medical Acupuncture Society, 20* (2-3), 82-99.

Cataldo, C.B., DeBruyne, L.K., & Whitney, E.N. (2003). *Nutrition and diet therapy principles and practice* (6th ed.). Belmont, CA: Wadsworth Publishing Company.

Cech, R.E. (2002). Guided imagery and music. *Share Guide, 64,* 30-32.

Centers for Disease Control and Prevention (CDC). (2013). *Healthy eating for a healthy weight.* http://www.cdc.gov/healthyweight/healthy_eating/index.html

Centers for Disease Control and Prevention (CDC). (2014a). *Unintentional drowning: Get the facts.* http://www.cdc.gov/HomeandRecreationalSafety/Water-Safety/water injuries-factsheet.html

Centers for Disease Control and Prevention (CDC). (2014b). *Obesity costs states billions in medical expenses.* http://www.cdc.gov/obesity/data/adult.html

Centers for Disease Control and Prevention (CDC). (2014c). *Overweight and obesity.* http://www.cdc.gov/obesity/index.html

Cerrato, P.L. (1997). Herbal therapy: More than just folklore. *RN, 60*(8), 51-53.

Cerrato, P.L. (1998). Aromatherapy: Is it for real? *RN, 61*(6), 51-52.

Chairman's Summary of the Conference, Education of Health Professionals in Complementary/Alternative Medicine, Josiah Macy, Jr. Foundation, 44 East 64th Street, New York, NY 10021.

Cherkin, D.C., Sherman, K.J., Deyo, R.A., & Shekelle, P.G. (2003). A review of the evidence for the effectiveness, safety, and cost of acupuncture, massage therapy, and spinal manipulation for back pain. *Annals of Internal Medicine, 138*(11), 898-906.

Cheung, Y.L., Molassiotis, A., & Chang, A.M. (2003). The effect of progressive muscle relaxation training on anxiety and quality of life after stoma surgery in colorectal cancer patients. *Psycho-Oncology, 12*(3), 254-66.

Chipfakacha, V.G. (1997). STD/HIV/AIDS knowledge, beliefs and practice of traditional healers in Botswana. *AIDS Care, 9*(4), 417-425.

Christensen, A. (2003). *Vegetarian diet and health.* http://americanyogaassociation.org/Diet%20main.html

Cocks, M. & Dold, A. (2000). The role of "African chemists" in the health care system of the Eastern Cape province of South Africa. *Social Science & Medicine, 51*(10), 1505-1515.

Coffey, M. (1999). Stress and burnout in forensic community mental health nurses: An investigation of its causes and effects. *Journal of Psychiatric and Mental Health Nursing, 6*(6), 433-43.

Cohen, K. (1998). Native American medicine. *Alternative Therapies in Health and Medicine, 4*(6), 45-57.

Cohen, S.M., Rousseau, M.E., & Robinson, E.H. (2000). Therapeutic use of selected herbs. *Holistic Nursing Practice, 14*(3), 59-68.

Colin, E. (1997). Sun salutation: Increasing your energy level. *Holistic Health News, 5*(6), 4-6.

Collins, N. & Navarre, A. (2003). Managing nutrition in an acutely ill patient. *Nursing, 33*(5), 32HN6-7.

Courtright, P. (1995). Eye care knowledge and practices among Malawian traditional healers and the development of collaborative blindness prevention programmes. *Social Science & Medicine, 41*(11), 1569-75.

Craig, G. (2000). *Therapeutic touch: Emotional Freedom Technique (EFT).* Accessed online February 2005, from http://www.therapeutic-touch.com

Crawford, C.C., Sparber, A.G., & Jonas, W.B. (2003). A systematic review of the quality of research on hands-on and distance healing: Clinical and laboratory studies. *Alternative Therapies in Health and Medicine, 9*(3 Suppl), A96-104.

Dallender, J., Nolan, P., Soares, J., & Thomsen, S., & Arnetz, B. (1999). A comparative study of the perceptions of British mental health nurses and psychiatrists of their work environment. *Journal of Advanced Nursing, 29*(1), 36-43.

Dash, M., Jackson, J., & Rasor, S. (1997). *Hidden wholeness: An African American spirituality for individuals and communities.* Cleveland, OH: United Church Press.

Dattilo, J. (2000). *Facilitation techniques in therapeutic recreation.* State College, PA: Venture Publishing, Inc.

Deatcher, J. (2002). Use of prayer in diabetes self-management. *Diabetes Educator, 28*(3), 390-4.

DeMarco-Sinatra, J. (2000). Relaxation training as a holistic nursing intervention. *Holistic Nursing Practice, 14*(3), 30-39.

Doherty, M.J., Wilensky, A.J., Holmes, M.D., Lewis, D.H., Rae, J., & Cohn, G.H. (2002). Singing seizures. *Neurology, 59*(9), 1435-38.

Donaldson, D. (2002). Herbal therapy, conventional drugs and quality control. *Journal of the Royal Society of Health, 122*(4), 209.

Dossey, B.M. (1998). Holistic modalities & healing moments. *American Journal of Nursing, 98*(6), 44-47.

Dossey, B.M. (1999). Barbara Dossey, RN, MS on holistic nursing, Florence Nightingale, and healing rituals. *Alternative Therapies in Health and Medicine, 5*(1), 78-86.

Dossey, B.M. (2001). Holistic nursing: Taking your practice to the next level. *Nursing Clinics of North America, 36*(1), 1-22.

Dossey, B.M. & Dossey, L. (1998). Body-mind-spirit: Attending to holistic care. *American Journal of Nursing, 98*(8), 35-38.

Dossey, B.M., Keegan, L., & Guzzetta, C.E. (Eds.). (2000). *Holistic nursing: A handbook for practice* (3rd ed.). Gaithersburg, MD: Aspen Publishers.

Dossey, L. (1993). *Healing words: The power of prayer and the practice of medicine.* San Francisco: Harper.

Dossey, L. (2000). Prayer and medical science: A commentary on the prayer study by Harris et al. and a response to critics. *Archives of Internal Medicine, 160*(12), 1735-37.

Dossey, L. (2003). Therapeutic touch at the crossroads: Observations on the Rosa study. *Alternative Therapies in Health and Medicine, 9*(1), 38-39.

Dull, H. (2004). *Watus: Freeing the body in water.* Victoria, BC, Canada: Trafford Publishing.

Dumas, H. & Francesconi, S. (2001). Aquatic therapy in pediatrics: Annotated bibliography. *Physical & Occupational Therapy in Pediatrics, 20*(4), 63-78.

Dung, H.C. (1995). Acupuncture points. *American Journal of Chinese Medicine, 13*(1-4), 49-64.

DuToit, B. (1998). Modern folk medicine in South Africa. *South African Journal of Ethnology, 21*(4), 145-53.

Dyson, P. (2002). Nutrition and diabetes control: Advise for non-dietitians. *British Journal of Community Nursing, 7*(8), 414-19.

Edwards, D. & Burnard, P. (2003). A systematic review of stress and stress management interventions for mental health nurses. *Journal of Advanced Nursing, 42*(2), 169-200.

Egan, K. & Arnold, R. (2003). Grief and bereavement care. *American Journal of Nursing, 103*(9), 42-52.

Eisenberg, D.M., Davis, R.B., Ettner, S.L., Appel, S., Wilkey, S., Van Rompay, M., et al. (1998). Trends in alternative medicine use in the United States, 1990-1997: Results of a follow-up national survey. *Journal of the American Medical Association, 280*(18), 1569-75.

Eliopoulos, C. (2004). *Invitation to holistic health: A guide to living a balanced life.* Boston: Jones & Bartlett.

Elliott, H. (2003). Imagework as a means for healing and personal transformation. *Complementary Therapies in Nursing and Midwifery, 9*(3), 118-124.

Emmerson, A.M. (2001). Emerging waterborne infections in health-care settings. *Emerging Infectious Diseases, 7*(2). http://wwwnc.cdc.gov/eid/article/7/2/70-0272_article

Enig, M. (1999). *Coconut: In support of good health in the 21st century.* Presented at the Asian Pacific Coconut Community's 36th Session, 1999. http://www.coconutoil.com/coconut_oil_21st_century.htm

Enig, M.G. & Fallon, S. (1998). The oiling of America (Part 1 of 2). *Nexus Magazine, Part 1, 6*(1), 7.

Evans, D. (2001). Music as an intervention in hospitals patients: A systematic review. *Best Practice, 5*(4), 1-6.

Federal Trade Commission (FTC). (2012). *Weighing the claims in diet ads.* http://www.consumer.ftc.gov/articles/0061-weighing-claims-diet-ads

Fellowes, D., Barnes, K., & Wilkinson, S. (2004). Aromatherapy and massage for symptom relief in patients with cancer. *The Cochrane Database of Systemic Reviews,* Issue 3. Art No.: CD002287.pub2. Chichester, UK: John Wiley & Sons, Ltd.

Fenton, M. (2003). Therapeutic touch: A nursing practice. *Alternative Therapies in Health and Medicine, 9*(1), 34-36.

Field, T. (2000). *Touch therapy.* Philadelphia: Churchill Livingstone.

Fife, B. (1999). *Saturated fat may save your life.* Colorado Springs, CO: Healthwise Publications.

Fife, B. (2000). *The healing miracles of coconut oil.* Colorado Springs, CO: Healthwise Publications.

Flaherty, J.H., Takahashi, R., Teoh, J., Kim, J.I., Habib, S., Ito, M., et al. (2001). Use of alternative therapies in older outpatients in the United States and Japan: Prevalence, reporting patterns, and perceived effectiveness. *Journal of Gerontology, 56*(10), M650-55.

Flanagan, K. (2001). Preoperative assessment: Safety considerations for patients taking herbal products. *Journal of Perianesthesia Nursing, 16*(1), 19-26.

Flemming, K. (2000). Review: Aromatherapy massage is associated with small, transient reductions in anxiety. *Evidence-Based Nursing, 3*(4), 118.

Fontane, K. (2000). *Healing practice: Alternative therapies for nursing.* Upper Saddle River, NJ: Prentice Hall.

Frank, D.I., Stephens, B., & Lee, S.H. (1998). Health promotion behaviours of African-American rural woman. *Clinical Excellence For Nurse Practitioners, 2*(3), 159-65.

Frass, M., Strassl, R. P., Friehs, H., Mullner, M., Kundi, M., Kaye, A. D. (2012). Use and acceptance of complementary and alternative medicine among the general population and medical personnel: A systematic review. *Ochsner Journal, 12*(1), 45-46.

Gallagher, L.M., Huston, M.J., Nelson, K.A., Walsh, D., & Steele, A.L. (2001). Music therapy in palliative medicine. *Supportive Care in Cancer, 9*(3), 156-61.

Gardner, M. (2003). The magic of therapeutic touching. *The Skeptical Inquire, 24*(6), 48-51.

Garfinkel, M.S., Singhal, A., Katz, W.A., Allan, D.A., Reshetar, R., & Schumacher, H.R., Jr. (1998). Yoga-based intervention for carpal tunnel syndrome: A randomized trial. *Journal of the American Medical Association, 280*(18), 1601-03.

Garfinkel, M. & Schumacher, H.R., Jr. (2000). Yoga. *Rheumatic Diseases Clinics of North America, 26*(1), 125-32.

Geary, A. (2000). Food and mood: A complementary treatment for mental health problems. *Positive Health, 56,* 30-34.

George, M. & Minski, R. (1996). Complementary therapy + high tech care. Interview by Susan Hudson. *Australian Nursing Journal, 4*(4), 34-36.

Gill, G.V., Redmond, S., Garratt, F., & Paisey, R. (1994). Diabetes and alternative medicine: Cause for concern. *Diabetes Medicine, 11*(2), 210-13.

Ginton, B. (1997). *The art of healing: Massage therapy.* http://www.qwl.com/mtwc/articles/mtart.html

Goldman, R.D. & Koren, G. (2003). Taking St. John's wort during pregnancy. *Canadian Family Physician, 49*(1), 29-30.

Good, M., Stanton-Hicks, M., Grass, J.A., Anderson, G.C., Lai, H.L., Roykulcharoen, V., et al. (2001). Relaxation and music to reduce postsurgical pain. *Journal of Advanced Nursing, 33*(2), 208-15.

Gozum, S. & Unsal, A. (2004). Use of herbal therapies by older, community-dwelling women. *Journal of Advanced Nursing, 46*(2), 171-78.

Graves, D.L., Shue, C.K., & Arnold, L. (2002). The role of spirituality in patient care: Incorporating spirituality training into medical school curriculum. *Academic Medicine: Journal of the Association of American Medical Colleges, 77*(11), 1167.

Greene, E. (2000). Massage therapy. In D. Novey (Ed.), *Clinicians complete reference to complementary and alternative medicine.* St. Louis: Mosby, pp. 338-348.

Griffiths, V. (2000). Traditional Chinese medicine: A case of dysmenorrhoea. *Australian Journal of Holistic Nursing, 7*(1), 42-3.

Harbin School of Healing Arts. (2014). http://harbinschoolofhealingarts.org/0010_Home.html

Hardwick, S. & Jordan S. (2002). Issues and innovations in nursing education. *Journal of Advanced Nursing, 38*(5), 524-35.

Harkness, E.F., Abbot, N.C., & Ernst, E. (2000). A randomized clinical trial of distance healing for peripheral common warts. *Journal of Medicine, 108*(6), 444-52.

Harper, C. (2001). The healing power of music. *Positive Health, 68*, 12-13.

Harris, W.S., Gowda, M., Kolb, J.W., Strychacz, C.P., Vacek, J.L., Jones, P.G., et al. (1999). A randomized, controlled trial of the effects of remote, intercessory prayer on outcomes in patients admitted to the coronary care unit. *Archives of Internal Medicine, 159*(19), 2273-78.

Haun, M., Mainous, R.O., & Looney, S.W. (2001). Effects of music on anxiety of women awaiting breast biopsy. *Journal of Behavioral Medicine, 27*(3), 127-32.

Hawk, C. (2000). *Therapeutic Touch: A healing lifestyle.* http://www.therapeutictouch.com/tt1.html

Healing Touch International. (1998). *What is healing touch?* http://www.healingtouch international.org

Heather, S. (2001). The healing power of sound. *Positive Health, 64*, 17-21.

Hilderbrandt, E. (1997). Have I angered my ancestors? Influences of culture on health care for elderly Black South Africans as an example. *Journal of Multicultural Nursing and Health, 3*(1), 40-49.

Hinds, C. (1997). Christie Hinds's personal crusade fighting AIDS with faith, facts & friendship. Interview by Karen Schmidt. *Journal of Christian Nursing, 14*(3), 19-22.

Hodes, R. (1997). Cross-cultural medicine and diverse health beliefs: Ethiopians abroad. *Western Journal of Medicine, 166*(1), 29-36.

Hoffman, H.G., Patterson, D.R., Magula, J., Carrougher, G.J., Zeltzer, K., Dagadakis, S. et al. (2004). Water-friendly virtual reality pain control during wound care. *Journal of Clinical Psychology, 60*(2), 189-95.

Holistic-online.com. (n.d.-a). *Acupuncture.* http://holistic-online.com/Acupuncture/acp_home.htm

Holistic-online.com. (n.d.-b). *Aromatherapy.* http://holistic-online.com/Aromatherapy/hol_aroma.htm

Holistic-online.com. (n.d.-c). *Herbal medicine.* http://holistic-online.com/Herbal-Med/hol_herb.htm

Holistic-online.com. (n.d.-d). *Hydrotherapy.* http://holistic-online.com/hydrotherapy.htm

Holistic-online.com. (n.d.-e). *Yoga.* http://holistic-online.com/Yoga/hol_yoga_breath_home.htm

Holmes, C., Hopkins, V., Hensford, C., MacLaughlin, V., Wilkinson, D., & Rosenvinge, H. (2002). Lavender oil as a treatment for agitated behaviour in severe dementia: A placebo controlled study. *International Journal of Geriatric Psychiatry, 17*(4), 305-08.

Holt, R.D. (1996). Review of species diversity in space and time by Rosenweig. *Quarterly Review of Biology and Evolution, 71*, 568.

Homsy, J., Katabira, E., Kabatesi, D., Mubiru, F., Kwamya, L., Tusaba, C., et al. (1999). Evaluating herbal medicine for the management of herpes zoster in human immuno-deficiency virus-infected patients in Kampala, Uganda. *Journal of Alternative and Complementary Medicine, 5*(6), 553-65.

Huebscher, R. & Shuler, P.A. (2003). *Natural, alternative, and complementary health care practices.* St. Louis: Mosby.

Hung-Youn, C. (1999). Cultural interbreeding between Korean Shamanism and imported religions. *Diogenes, 47*(3), 50-62.

International Academy of Advance Reflexology. (2003). *Reflexology accurately defined.* http://www.reflexology-research.com

International Institute of Reflexology. (n.d.-a). *Facts about reflexology.* http://www.reflexology-usa.net/facts.htm

International Institute of Reflexology. (n.d.-b). *The Ingham method of reflexology.* http://www.reflexology-usa.net

Jacobs, B.P., Mehling, W., Avins, A.L., Goldberg, H.A., Acree, M., Lasater, J.H., et al. (2004). Feasibility of conducting a clinical trial on Hatha yoga for chronic low back pain: Methodological lessons. *Alternative Therapies in Health and Medicine, 10*(2), 80-83.

Jellin, J., Gregory, P., Batz, F., Hitchens, K., et al. (2000). *Natural medicines comprehensive database* (4th ed.). Stockton, CA: Therapeutic Research Faculty.

Jonas, W.B. & Crawford, C.C. (2003). Science and spiritual healing: A critical review of spiritual healing, "energy" medicine, and intentionality. *Alternative Therapies in Health and Medicine, 9*(2), 56-61.

Jones, P.J. (1997). Regulation of cholesterol biosynthesis by diet in humans. *American Journal of Clinical Nutrition, 66*(2), 438-46.

Kacperek, L. (1997). Patients' views on the factors which would influence the use of an aromatherapy massage out-patient service. *Complementary Therapies in Nursing and Midwifery, 3*(2), 51-7.

Karr, W. (1998). Music to heal: Tonic from tones and remedies from rhythms. *WE Magazine, 2*(6), 52-54.

Keegan, L. (1998). Getting comfortable with alternative and complementary modalities. *Nursing, 98,* 50-53.

Keegan, L. (2000). Alternative and complementary modalities for managing stress and anxiety. *Critical Care Nurse, 23*(3), 93-96.

Keegan, L. (2003). Therapies to reduce stress and anxiety. *Critical Care Nursing Clinics of North America, 15*(3), 321-27.

Keegan, L. & Keegan, G.T. (1998). *Healing waters: The miraculous health benefits of Earth's most essential resources.* New York: Berkley Books.

Kelly, A.L. (2002). Prayer in a petri dish? *Health, 16*(10), 46.

Kelly, L. (1994). Historical use of therapeutic activity in Africa. *South African Journal of Occu-pa-tional Therapy, 24*(2), 26-30.

Kelly, L. (1995). What occupational therapists can learn from traditional healers. *British Journal of Occupational Therapy, 58*(3), 111-14.

Khalsa, D.S. (2000). Medical meditations. *Total Health, 22*(4), 59-61.

Kiefer, D., Shah, S., Gardiner, P., & Wechkin, H. (2001). Finding information on herbal therapy: A guide to useful sources for clinicians. *Alternative Therapies in Health and Medicine, 7*(6), 74-78.

Kilfedder, C.J., Power, K.G., & Wells, T.J. (2001). Burnout in psychiatric nursing. *Journal of Advanced Nursing, 34*(3), 383-96.

Kleiner, C. (2002). Mind-body fitness: Yoga booms in popularity as a way to heighten flexibility, improve breathing, and gain sanity. *U.S. News & World Report, 132*(16), 53-55.

Kogut, V. (2001). Complementary and alternative dietary therapies. *Clinical Journal of Oncology Nursing, 5*(6), 283-86.

Konlian, C. (1999). Aquatic therapy: Making a wave in the treatment of low back injuries. *Orthopedic Nursing, 18*(1), 11-18.

Kozier, B., Erb, G., Berman, A.J., & Burke, K. (2000). *Fundamentals of nursing: Concepts, process, and practice* (6th ed.). Upper Saddle River, NJ: Prentice Hall Health.

Krieger, D. (1974). Healing by the laying-on of hands as a facilitator of bioenergetics change: the response of in-vivo human hemoglobin. *Psycho-energy systems, 1,* 121.

Krieger, D. (1979). *Therapeutic touch: How to use your hands to help or to heal.* Englewood Cliffs, NJ: Prentice Hall.

Krieger, D. (1998). Dolores Krieger, RN, PhD, healing with therapeutic touch. Interview by Bonnie Horrigan. *Alternative Therapies in Health and Medicine, 4*(1), 86-92.

Krieger, D. (1999). Should nurses practice therapeutic touch? Should nursing schools teach therapeutic touch? *Journal of Professional Nursing, 15*(3), 200-01.

Kuhn, M. (1999). *Complementary therapies for health care providers.* Philadelphia: Lippincott.

Kunz, B. & Kunz, K. (2004). *Reflexology certification.* http://www.foot-reflexologist.com/education.htm

Kunz, B. & Kunz, K. (2005). *Interactive footmap.* http://uk.dk.com/static/cs/uk/11/features/reflexology/extract.html

Kusmirek, J. (1998). Down to basics: The question of base gels and creams for aromatherapy. Interview by Caroline Stevensen. *Complementary Therapies in Nursing and Midwifery, 4*(4), 118-19.

Labarthe, D. & Ayala, C. (2002). Nondrug interventions in hypertension prevention and control. *Cardiology Clinics, 20*(2), 249-63.

Lao, L., Hamilton, G.R., Fu, J., & Berman, B.M. (2003). Is acupuncture safe? A systematic review of case reports. *Alternative Therapies in Health and Medicine, 9*(1), 72-83.

Larkin, M. (2001). Music tunes up memory in dementia patients. *Lancet, 357*(9249), 47-49.

Laurion, S. (2003). The effect of two nursing interventions on the postoperative outcomes of gynecologic laparoscopic patients. *Journal of Perianesthesia Nursing, 18*(4), 254-61.

Ledwith, S.P. (1995). Therapeutic touch and mastectomy: A case study. *RN, 58*(7), 51-53.

Lee, L. (1999). Introducing herbal medicine into conventional health care settings. *Journal of Nurse-Midwifery, 44*(3), 253-66.

Lee, A.C. & Kemper, K.J. (2000). Practice patterns of massage therapists. *Journal of Alternative and Complementary Medicine, 6*(6), 527-29.

Lee, J.S., Kawakubo, K., & Kawamura, H. (2003). Assessment of worksite health promotion environments. *Journal of Occupational Health [Japan], 45*(2), 57-66.

Lewis, K. (1998). The Bonny Method of guided personal imagery and music: Matrix for transpersonal experience. *Journal of the Association of Music and Imagery, 6,* 63-86.

Lewis, M. (May 2000). Why music heals your mind. Interview. *Sunday Express, page 51, 21.*

Lilley, L.L. & Aucker, R.S. (2001). *Pharmacology and the nursing process* (3rd ed.). St. Louis: Mosby.

Lock, S., Dunea, G., Last, J., Walton, J., Beeson, P., & Barondess, J. (2001). *Oxford Illustrated Companion of Medicine.* United Kingdon: Oxford University Press.

Lowdermilk, D.L. & Perry, S.E. (2004). *Maternity & women's health care* (8th ed.). St. Louis: Mosby.

Lower, J.S., Bonsack, C., Guion, J. (2003). Peace and quiet. *Nursing Management, 34*(4), 40A-40D.

Lowry, L.W. & Conco, D. (2002). Exploring the meaning of spirituality with aging adults in Appalachia. *Journal of Holistic Nursing, 20*(4), 388-402.

Luskin, F. (2000). Review of the effect of spiritual and religious factors on mortality and morbidity with a focus on cardiovascular and pulmonary disease. *Journal of Cardiopulmonary Rehabilitation, 20*(1), 8-15.

Luskin, F.M., Newell, K.A., Griffith, M., Holmes, M., Telles, S., DiNucci, E., et al. (2000). A review of mind/body therapies in the treatment of musculoskeletal disorders with implications for the elderly. *Alternative Therapies in Health and Medicine, 6*(2), 46-56.

Luskin, F.M., Newell, K.A., Griffith, M., Holmes, M., Telles, S., Marvasti, F.F., et al. (1998). A review of mind-body therapies in the treatment of cardiovascular disease. Part 1: Implications for the elderly. *Alternative Therapies in Health and Medicine, 4*(3), 46-61.

Lutz, C.A. & Przytulski, K.R. (2001). *Nutrition and diet therapy* (3rd ed.). Philadelphia: F.A. Davis Co.

Lutz, E.R. (1999). Watsu-aquatic body work. *Beginning, 19*(2), 9-11.

Mackereth, P. & Wright, J. (1997). Therapeutic touch: Nursing activity or form of spiritual healing? *Complementary Therapies in Nursing and Midwifery, 3*(4), 106-10.

Mackey, B.T. (2001). Massage therapy and reflexology awareness. *Nursing Clinics of North America, 36*(1), 159-70.

Macrae, J. (1988). *Therapeutic touch: A practical guide.* New York: Knopf.

Malhotra, V., Singh, S., Tandon, O.P., Madhu, S.V., Prasad, A., & Sharma, S.B. (2002). Effect of yoga asanas on nerve conduction in type 2 diabetes. *Indian Journal of Physiology and Pharmacology, 46*(3), 298-306.

Mann, E. (2003) Managing pain: Integrative approaches to pain management. *BMJ, 326*(14), 1320-24.

Manocha, R. (2003). Sahaja yoga in asthma. *Thorax, 58*(9), 825-26.

Marley, J.E., Searle, P., Chamberlain, N.L., Turnbull, D.R., & Leahy, C.M. (2001). Carols in the wind. *Medical Journal of Australia, 175*(11-12), 656-58.

Martin, M. (2000). Reflexology: What is its true potential? *Positive Health, 53,* 18-22.

Martin, M. (2001). The art and science of reflexology: The vital link. *Positive Health, 64,* 22-23.

Massagetherapy.com. (n.d.). *Types of massage and bodywork defined.* http://www.massage therapy.com/glossary/index.php#r

Mattie, J. (2000). African American women's definition of spirituality and religiosity. *Journal of Black Psychology, 26*(1), 101-122.

Mattie, J. (2001). Religion and African American political life. *Political Psychology, 22*(2), 263-78.

Mattie, J. & Jagers, R. (2001). A religional framework for the study of religiosity and spirituality in the lives of African Americans. *Journal of Community Psychology, 28*(5), 519-539.

Mazo, E. (2002). The medicine of music. *Health, 16*(5), 74-81.

Mazo, E. & Parker, M. (2002). The medicine of music. *Health,* June 2002:74. Academic Search Elite. EBSCO-Host database.

Mbiti, J.S. (1990). *African religions & philosophy.* London: Heinemann.

McCaffrey, R. (2000). The lived experience of listening to music while recovering from surgery. *Journal of Holistic Nursing, 4,* 378-390.

McCaffrey, R. & Fowler. (2003). Gigong practice: A pathway to health and healing. *Holistic Nursing Practice, 17*(2), 110-116.

McCaffrey, R. & Locsin, R. (2002). Music listening as a nursing intervention: A symphony of practice. *Holistic Nursing Practice, 16*(3), 70-77.

McCaffrey, R.G. & Good, M. (2000). The lived experience of listening to music while recovering from surgery. *Journal of Holistic Nursing, 18*(4), 378-90.

McIver, S., O'Halloran, P., & McGartland, M. (2004). The impact of Hatha yoga on smoking behavior. *Alternative Therapies in Health and Medicine, 10*(2), 22-23.

McLeod, T. (1997). Work stress among community psychiatric nurses. *British Journal of Nursing, 6*(10), 569-74.

McNeely, C. (1997). Childbirth educators and the use of touch modalities. *International Journal of Childbirth Education, 12*(4), 4-6.

Meraviglia, M.G. (1999). Critical analysis of spirituality and its empirical indicators: Prayer and meaning in life. *Journal of Holistic Nursing, 17*(1), 18-33.

Mentgen, J.L. (2001). Healing touch. *The Nursing Clinics of North America, 36*(1), 143-58.

Michalsen, A., Ludtke, R., Buhring, M., Spahn, G., Langhorst, J., & Dobos, G.J. (2003). Thermal hydrotherapy improves quality of life and hemodynamic function in patients with chronic heart failure. *American Heart Journal, 146*(4), E11.

Micozzi, M. (2001). *Fundamentals of Complementary and Alternative Medicine.* New York: Churchill Livingstone.

Miller, W.C. (2001). Effective diet and exercise treatment for overweight and recommendation interventions. *Sports Medicine, 31*(10), 717-24.

Molloy, C. (2000). Touch therapy. *Massage and Bodywork, 15*(6), 12-23.

Morrison, E.F. & Thornton, K.A. (1999). Influence of southern spiritual beliefs on perceptions of mental illness. *Issues in Mental Health Nursing, 20*(5), 443-58.

Mystic World Fellowship. (1999). *The eight main yogas.* http://www.yogaworld.org/yogas.htm

Nagai-Jacobson, M.G. & Burkhardt, M.A. (1989). Spirituality: Cornerstone of holistic nursing practice. *Holistic Nursing Practice, 3*(3), 18-26.

Nagai-Jacobson, M.G. & Burkhardt, M.A. (1996). Viewing persons as stories: A perspective for holistic care. *Alternative Therapy, 2*(4), 54-58.

Nagai-Jacobson, M.G. & Burkhardt, M.A. (2001). Nurturing and caring for self. *Nursing Clinics of North America, 36*(1), 23-32.

National Association For Holistic Aromatherapy (NAHA). (2014a). *What is aromatherapy?* http://www.naha.org/explore-aromatherapy/about-aromatherapy/what-is-aromatherapy/

National Association for Holistic Aromatherapy (NAHA). (2014b). *Methods of Application.* http://www.naha.org/explore-aromatherapy/about-aromatherapy/methods-of-application

National Association for Holistic Aromatherapy. (2014c). *Most commonly used essential oils.* http://www.naha.org/explore-aromatherapy/about-aromatherapy/most-commonly-used-essential-oils

National Center for Complementary and Alternative Medicine (NCCAM). (2014a). http://nccam.nih.gov/about

National Center for Complementary and Alternative Medicine. (2014b). *What is complementary and alternative medicine (CAM)?* http://nccam.nih.gov/health/whatiscam/index.htm

National Center for Complementary and Alternative Medicine. (2014c). *NCCAM funding: Appropriations history.* http://nccam.nih.gov/about/budget/appropriations.htm

National Institutes of Health (NIH). (n.d.). Office of Dietary Supplements (ODS) – *Dietary Supplement Fact Sheets.* http://ods.od.nih.gov/factsheets/list-all/

National Institutes of Health (NIH). (1994). Office of Dietary Supplements (ODS) – *Dietary Supplement Health and Education Act of 1994.* http://ods.od.nih.gov/pdf/About/DSHEA_Wording.aspx.pdf

National Institutes of Health (NIH). (2011). Office of Dietary Supplements (ODS) – *Botanical Dietary Supplements,* http://ods.od.nih.gov/factsheets/BotanicalBackground-HealthProfessional/

National Institutes of Health (NIH). (2014a). National Center for Complementary and Alternative Medicine (NCCAM) – *Complementary, alternative, or integrative health: What's in a name?* http://nccam.nih.gov/health/whatiscam

National Institutes of Health (NIH). (2014b). National Center for Complementary and Alternative Medicine (NCCAM) – *Using dietary supplements wisely.* http://nccam.nih.gov/health/supplements/wiseuse.htm

National Institutes of Health (NIH). (2012). National Cancer Institute – *Aroma therapy and essential oils.* http://www.cancer.gov/cancertopics/pdq/cam/aromatherapy/patient/Page2#Section_45

National Institutes of Health (NIH). (2013). National Center for Complementary and Alternative Medicine (NCCAM) – *Traditional chinese medicine: An introduction.* http://nccam.nih.gov/health/whatiscam/chinesemed.htm

National Institutes of Health (NIH). (2014c). National Center for Complementary and Alternative Medicine (NCCAM) – *Acupuncture may be helpful for chronic pain: A meta-analysis.* http://nccam.nih.gov/research/results/spotlight/091012

Natural Holistic Health. (2012). *Single Essential Oil Profiles, Benefits, Indications,* http://www.natural-holistic-health.com/single-essential-oil-profiles

Nelson, N.J. (1997). Scents or nonsense: Aromatherapy's benefits still subject to debate. *Journal of the National Cancer Institute, 89*(18), 1334-36.

Newlin, K., Knafl, K., & Melkus, G.D. (2002). African-American spirituality: A concept analysis. *Advances in Nursing Science, 25*(2), 57-70.

Newshan, G. & Schuller-Civitella, D. (2003). Large clinical study shows value of therapeutic touch program. *Holistic Nursing Practice, 17*(4), 189-92.

Nightingale, F. (1859). *Notes on nursing: What it is and what it is not.* London: Harrison. Reprinted by Lippincott, 2001.

Nirmala-Dharm, V. (2013). *Chakras and the channels of energy.* http://www.sahajayoga.org/ChakrasAndSubtlebody

Ntuli, P.B. (1997). Study to discover the influence and effects of non-medical practitioners on black terminally ill patients in Edendale, Pietermaritzburg. *South African Journal of Nursing, 20*(1), 60.

Nurse Healers-Professional Associates International. (2014). *Therapeutic touch.* http://therapeutic-touch.org

Odebiyi, A.I. (1989). Food taboos in maternal and child health: The views of traditional healers in Ile-Ife, Nigeria. *Social Science & Medicine, 28*(9), 985-96.

Ogaga, A. (1999). Special herbal complex for women. *Healthcare, 14*(6), 13.

Ogdin, C., Carroll, M., Kit, B., & Flegal, K. (2014). Prevalence of Childhood and Adult Obesity in the United States, 2011-2012. *The Journal of the American Medical Association (JAMA), 311*(8). http://jama.jamanetwork.com/article.aspx?articleid=1832542

O'Kelly, J. (2002). Music therapy in palliative care: Current perspectives. *International Journal of Palliative Nursing, 8*(3), 130-136.

Olsson, H., Backe, H., Sorensen, S., & Kock, M. (2002). The essence of humour and its effects and functions: A qualitative study. *Journal of Nursing Management, 10*(1), 21-26.

Organic Facts. (2014). *Health benefits of coconut oil.* https://www.organicfacts.net/organic-oils/organic-coconut-oil/health-benefits-of-coconut-oil.html

Osborn, K. (2003). Sea of calm: Water therapy touches young spirit. *Massage and Body Works, Feb/March,* 44-48.

Ovechkin, A., Lee, S.M., & Kim, K.S. (2001). Thermovisual evaluation of acupuncture points. *Acupuncture and Electro-Therapeutics Research, 26*(1-2), 11-23.

Pal, S.K. & Shukla, Y. (2003). Herbal medicine: Current status and the future. *Asian Pacific Journal of Cancer Prevention, 4*(4), 281-88.

Paterson, J.G. & Zderad, L.T. (1988). *Humanistic nursing.* New York: National League for Nursing.

Patterson, E.F. (1998). The philosophy and physics of holistic health care: Spiritual healing as a workable interpretation. *Journal of Advanced Nursing, 27*(2), 287-93.

Payne, K. (1997). Creating a home yoga practice. *Holistic Health News, 5*(6), 4-6.

Pellitteri, J. (2000). The consultant corner. Music therapy in special educational settings: Psychological aspects. *Journal of Educational and Psychological Consultation, 11*(3), 379-92.

Perez, C. (2003). Clinical aromatherapy. Part 1: An introduction into nursing practice. *Clinical Journal of Oncology Nursing, 7*(5), 595-596.

Peterson, C. (2001). Exercise in 94° F water for a patient with multiple sclerosis. *Physical Therapy, 81*(4), 1049-1058.

Pinn, G. (2001). Herbal medicine. What is the evidence? *Australian Family Physician, 30*(12), 1154-1159.

Pinn, G. & Pallett, L. (2002). Herbal medicine in pregnancy. *Complementary Therapies in Nursing and Midwifery, 8*(2), 77-80.

Plaskin, G. (2002). Why laughter is good for you. *Family Circle, 115*(3), 38.

Popoola, M.M. (2000a). Paradigm shift: A clarion call for a holistic to chronic wound management. *Advances in Skin & Wound Care, 13*(1), 47-48.

Popoola, M.M. (2000b). *Where in Africa? A cultural saga from Denver to Lagos.* Lagos, Nigeria: Mace Books.

Popoola, M.M. (2003a). Complementary therapy in chronic wound management: A holistic caring case study and praxis model. *Holistic Nursing Practice, 17*(3), 152-58.

Popoola, M.M. (2003b). From descriptive survey to a caring healing praxis model of chronic wound management. *West African Journal of Nursing, 14*(1), 13-21.

Popoola, M.M. & Clinton, M. (2004). Diabetes: A spiritual glimpse. *West African Journal of Nursing, 15*(1), 42-47.

Prins, J. & Cutner, D. (1999). Aquatic therapy in the rehabilitation of athletic injuries. *Clinics in Sports Medicine, 18*(2), 447-61.

Rajagopal, D., Mackenzie, E., Bailey, C., & Lavizzo-Mourey, R. (2002). The effectiveness of spiritual-based intervention to alleviate subsyndromal anxiety and minor depression among older adults. *Journal of Religions and Health, 41*(2), 153-166.

Ram, F.S., Holloway, E.A., & Jones, P.W. (2003). Breathing retraining for asthma. *Respiratory Medicine, 97*(5), 501-07.

Rankin-Box, D. (2001). *Nurses' handbook of complementary therapies* (2nd ed.). London: Bailliere-Tindall.

Rankin-Box, D. (2002). Ethics and quality in complementary therapy education. *Nursing Times, 98*(2), 40-42.

Rankin-Box, D. & Campbell, K. (2000). Is there a rational basis underlying alternative medicine? *Nursing Times, 96*(23), 18.

Reflexology Association of America (RAA). (2011). *RAA's definition of reflexology.* http://reflexology-usa.org/information/raas-definition-of-reflexology

Reflexology Association of America (RAA). (2014a). *Our history.* http://reflexology-usa.org/information/our-history

Reflexology Association of America (RAA). (2014b). *Standards and ethics.* http://reflexology-usa.org/information/standards-and-ethics

Reflexology Association of America (RAA). (2014c). *National Certification.* http://reflexology-usa.org/national-certification/

Richards, K., Nagel, C., Markie, M., Elwell, J., & Barone, C. (2003). Use of complementary and alternative therapies to promote sleep in critically ill patients. *Critical Care Nursing Clinics of North America, 15*(3), 329-40.

Ricks, S. (1995). *The reflexology workout: Hand & foot massage for super health & rejuvenation.* New York: Crow Trade Publication.

Ricks, S. (2001). Gentle touch of reflexology. *Positive Health, 67,* 26-31.

Ridgway, G.L. & Tedder, R.S. (1996). Birthing pools and infection control. *Lancet, 347*(9007), 1051-52.

Riley, D. (2004). Hatha yoga and the treatment of illness. *Alternative Therapies in Health and Medicine, 10*(2), 20-21.

Robinson, B. (2003). *Therapeutic touch studies.* http://www.religioustolerance.org/ther_tou2.htm

Rose, J. (1995). *The aromatherapy book: Application and inhalation.* North Atlantic, Berkeley.

Rose, J. (2001). Herbs and aromatherapy as anti-inflammatory. *Massage and Bodywork, 16*(2), 56-62.

Saeki, Y. (2000). The effect of foot-bath with or without the essential oil of lavender on the autonomic nervous system: A randomized trial. *Complementary Therapies in Medicine, 8*(1), 2-7.

Santa Ana, C.F. (2001). The adoption of complementary and alternative medicine by hospitals: A framework for decision-making. *Journal of Healthcare Management, 46*(4), 250-60.

Saper, R.B., Eisenberg, D.M., Davis, R.B., Culpepper, L., & Phillips, R.S. (2004). Prevalence and patterns of adult yoga use in the United States: Results of a national survey. *Alternative Therapies in Health and Medicine, 10*(2), 44-49.

Schaeffer, R. (1997). *Yoga for your spiritual muscles: A complete yoga program to strengthen body and spirit.* Wheaton, IL: Quest Books.

Schaeffer, R. (1999). Yoga notebook: Better health through movement. *Natural Health, 9*(9), 32.

Schaeffer, R. (2002a). Sharpen your memory with yoga. *Natural Health, 32*(6), 40-42.

Schaeffer, R. (2002b). Calm digestive upset with yoga. *Natural Health, 32*(5), 38-41.

Schaeffer, R. (2002c). Improve your workout with yoga. *Natural Health, 32*(4), 48.

Schaeffer, R. (2002d). Improve your posture with yoga. *Natural Health, 32*(2), 46-48.

Schaeffer, R. (2002e). Ease travel fatigue with yoga. *Alternative Health Watch – Natural Health, 32*(9), 52-54.

Schaeffer, R. (2002f). When pregnant, feel good with yoga. *Natural Health, 32*(8), 52-54.

Schiedermayer, D. (2000). Music therapy for the relief of postoperative pain. In *Physician's guide to alternative medicine,* Vol II (pp. 295-297). Atlanta: American Healthcare Consultant.

Schorr, J.A. (1993). Music and pattern change in chronic pain. *Advances in Nursing Science, 15*(4), 27-36.

Sharma, S.K. & Singh, B. (2000). *Yoga: A guide to healthy living.* New York: Lester Press Ltd., Forth Impress.

Sheler, J.L. (2001). Drugs, scalpel ... and faith? *U.S. News & World Report, 131*(1), 46.

Simon, H.B. (2004). Hot tub sense and safety. *Harvard Men's Health Watch, 8*(6), 8.

Skeptic's Dictionary. (1998). *Therapeutic touch.* http://skepdic.com/tt.html

Smith, B. (2001). Nontraditional choices. *Nursing 2001, 31*(9), 68.

Smith, M.C., Stallings, M.A., Mariner, S., & Burrall, M. (1999). Benefits of massage therapy for hospitalized patients: A descriptive and qualitative evaluation. *Alternative Therapies in Health and Medicine, 5*(4) 64-71.

Sova, R. (2004). The chi of water. *Rehab Management, 17*(3), 20-23.

Spence, J.E. & Olson, M.A. (1997). Quantitative research on therapeutic touch. An integrative review of the literature 1985-1995. *Scandinavian Journal of Caring Sciences, 11*(3), 183-90.

Stall, L. (2003, September 28). Rex and music. In *60 Minutes News Magazine.* New York: CBS Broadcasting Inc.

Steinberg, L. (2002). Yoga. In M.A. Bright (Ed.), *Holistic health and healing.* Philadelphia: F.A. Davis.

Stephenson, N.L. & Dalton, J.A. (2003). Using reflexology for pain management: A review. *Journal of Holistic Nursing, 21*(2), 179-91.

Stevenson, C. (1994). Aromatherapy: The essentials (continuing education credit). *Nursing Standard, 9*(9 Suppl Nu), 3-8.

Stevensen, C. (1995). Non-pharmacological aspects of acute pain management. *Complementary Therapies in Nursing and Midwifery, 1*(3), 77-84.

Stevensen, C.J. (1998). Aromatherapy in dermatology. *Clinics in Dermatology, 16*(6), 689-94.

Stone, J. (1999) Using complementary therapy within nursing – Some ethical and legal considerations. *Complementary Therapies in Nursing and Midwifery, 5*, 46-50.

Stone, J. (2001). How might traditional remedies be incorporated into discussions of integrated medicine? *Complementary Therapies in Nursing and Midwifery, 7*(2), 55-58.

Stone, J. (2002). Identifying ethicolegal and professional principles in reflexology. *Com-plementary Therapies in Nursing and Midwifery, 8*(4), 217-21.

Strang, S., Strang, P., & Ternestedt, B. (2002). Spiritual needs as defined by Swedish nursing staff. *Journal of Clinical Nursing 11*(1), 48-57.

Swedish Massage. (2003). *Swedish massage.* http://www.abmp.com

Szelenyi, I. & Brune, K. (2002). Herbal remedies for asthma treatment: Between myth and reality. *Drugs of Today, 38*(4), 265-303.

Taylor, E.J. (2003). Prayer's clinical issues and implications. *Holistic Nursing Practice, 17*(4), 179-88.

Taylor, E.J. & Outlaw, F.H. (2002). Use of prayer among persons with cancer. *Holistic Nursing Practice, 16*(3), 46-60.

Tella, A. (1999). The practice of traditional medicine in Africa. *Nigerian Medical Journal, 9*(5-6), 607-12.

Telepo, L. (1993). *International Academy of Advanced Reflexology: The Manuscript Introduction to Reflexology.* http://www. reflexology.net/about.htm

Thomas, D.V. (2002). Aromatherapy: Mythical, magical, or medicinal? *Holistic Nursing Practice, 16*(5), 8-16.

Thomas, K.J., Nicholl, J.P., & Coleman, P. (2001). Use and expenditure on complementary medicine in England: A population based survey. *Complementary Therapies in Medicine, 9*(1), 2-11.

Thornton, L. (2014). American Holistic Nurses Association – *What is holistic nursing?* http://www.ahna.org/About-Us/What-is-Holistic-Nursing

Torr, M.A. (2001). Meditation and psychotherapy: An effective combination. *Perspectives in Psychiatric Care, 37*(3), 103-06.

Townsend, J. (2001). Shamanism: Traditional and contemporary approaches to the mastery of spirits and healing. *American Anthropologist, 103*(1), 253-254.

Tsey, K. (1997). Traditional medicine in contemporary Ghana: A public policy analysis. *Social Science & Medicine, 45*(7), 1065-74.

Tuck, I., McCain, N.L., & Elswick, R.K., Jr. (2001). Spirituality and psychosocial factors in persons living with HIV. *Journal of Advanced Nursing, 33*(6), 776-83.

Tuck, I., Pullen, L., & Wallace, D. (2001). A comparative study of the spiritual perspectives and interventions of mental health and parish nurses. *Issues in Mental Health Nursing, 22*(6), 593-605.

Tuck, I., Wallace, D., & Pullen, L. (2001). Spirituality and spiritual care provided by parish nurses. *Western Journal of Nursing Research, 23*(5), 441-53.

Ulett, G.A., Han, J., & Han, S. (1998). Traditional and evidence-based acupuncture: History, mechanisms, and present status. *Southern Medical Journal, 91*(12), 1115-20.

Ulloth, J.K. (2002). The benefits of humor in nursing education. *Journal of Nursing Education, 41*(11), 476-81.

U.S. Consumer Product Safety Commission (CPSC). (2008). *The Pool and Spa Safety Act (P&SS Act)*. http://www.poolsafely.gov/pool-spa-safety-act/

United States Department of Agriculture (USDA). (2014). *Vitamins and Minerals*. http://fnic.nal.usda.gov/food-composition/vitamins-and-minerals

U.S. Department of Health and Human Services. (2000). *Healthy people 2010: Understanding and improving health*. Washington, DC: U.S. Government Printing Office.

U.S. Department of Health and Human Services. (2001). *The surgeon general's call to action to prevent and decrease overweight and obesity*. Washington, DC: U.S. Government Printing Office.

U.S. Food and Drug Administration (FDA), Center for Food Safety and Applied Nutrition (CFSAN). (2013). *National food safety programs*. http://www.fda.gov/AboutFDA/CentersOffices/OfficeofFoods/CFSAN/default.htm

U.S. Food and Drug Administration (FDA). (2013). CFR – Code of Federal Regulations Title 21(2007) – *Current Good Manufacturing Practice in Manufacturing, Packaging, Labeling, or Holding Operations for Dietary Supplements*. http://www.accessdata.fda.gov/scripts/cdrh/cfdocs/cfcfr/CFRSearch.cfm?CFRPart=111

U.S. Food and Drug Administration (FDA). (2014a). *Dietary Supplements: What You Need to Know*. http://www.fda.gov/Food/DietarySupplements/UsingDietarySupplements/ucm109760.htm

U.S. Food and Drug Administration (FDA). (2014b). *Dietary Supplements*. http://www.fda.gov/Food/DietarySupplements/default.htm

U.S. Food and Drug Administration (FDA). (2009). *Dietary Supplement Health and Education Act (DSHEA) of 1994*. http://www.fda.gov/regulatoryinformation/legislation/federalfooddrugandcosmeticactfdcact/significantamendmentstothefdcact/ucm148003.htm

U.S. National Library of Medicine. (2012). *Classics of traditional Chinese medicine: Yin and yang*. http://www.nlm.nih.gov/exhibition/chinesemedicine/yin_yang.html

University of Maryland Medical Center (UMM). (2013). *Massage*. http://umm.edu/health/medical/altmed/treatment/massage

Vanderbilt, S. (2001). A good foot rub: Easing cancer pain and anxiety. *Massage and Bodywork, 16*(3), 96-100.

Van Fleet, S. (2000). Relaxation and imagery for symptom management: Improving patient assessment and individualizing treatment. *Oncology Nursing Forum, 27*(3), 501-10.

Vass, S. (1989). *Laughing your way to good health*. Atlanta: HMR Publication Group, Inc.

Vender, R.B. (2003). Adverse reactions to herbal therapy in dermatology. *Skin Therapy Letter, 8*(3), 5-8.

Venes, D., (Ed.) (2013). *Taber's Cyclopedic Medical Dictionary* (22nd ed.). Philadelphia: F.A. Davis.

Vontress, C.F. (1999). Interview with a traditional African healer. *Journal of Mental Health Counseling, 21*(4), 326 - 337.

Wall, L.L. (2002). Fitsari 'dan Duniya. An African (Hausa) praise song about vesicovaginal fistulas. *Obstetrics and Gynecology, 100*(6), 1328-32.

Walton, J. (1999). Spirituality of patients recovering from an acute myocardial infarction: A grounded theory study. *Journal of Holistic Nursing, 17*(1), 34-53.

Walton, M.A., Blow, F.C., Bingham, C.R., & Chermack, S.T. (2003). Individual and social/environmental predictors of alcohol and drug use 2 years following substance abuse treatment. *Addictive Behaviors, 28*(4), 627-42.

Waterhouse, D. (1993). *Outsmarting the female fat cell: The first weight-control program designed specifically for women.* New York: Warner Books.

Webster, M. (2001). Shiatsu, nutrition and mind in the treatment of ME. *Positive Health, 66,* 49.

Webster, N. (1979). *Merriam-Webster's Collegiate dictionary* (8th ed.). Springfield, MA: G & C Merriam Company.

White, J.M. (2001). Music as intervention: A notable endeavor to improve patient outcomes. *Holistic Nursing Care, 36*(1), 83-91.

Whitehill, W. & Gustman, B. (2002). Massage and skin conditions: Indications and contraindications. *Athletic Therapy Today, 7*(3), 24-28.

White Lotus Foundation. (2014). http://www.whitelotus.org

Wiesendanger, H., Werthmuller, L., Reuter, K., & Walach, H. (2001). Chronically ill patients treated by spiritual healing improve in quality of life: Results of a randomized waiting-list controlled study. *Journal of Alternative and Complementary Medicine, 7*(1), 45-51.

Wilkinson, D., Gcabashe, L., & Lurie, M. (1999). Traditional healers as tuberculosis treatment supervisors: Precedent and potential. *International Journal of Tuberculosis Lung Disease, 3*(9), 838-42.

Wilkinson, D.S., Knox, P.L., Chatman, J.E., Johnson, T.L., Barbour, N., Myles, Y., et al. (2002). The clinical effectiveness of healing touch. *Journal of Alternative and Complementary Medicine, 8*(1), 33-47.

Winter, M.J., Paskin, S., Baker, T. (1994). Music reduces stress and anxiety of patients in the surgical holding area. *Journal of Postanesthesia Nursing, 9*(6), 340-43.

World Health Organization (WHO). (1998). *Regulatory situation of herbal medicines: A worldwide review.* http://apps.who.int/iris/bitstream/10665/63801/1/WHO_TRM_98.1.pdf?ua=1

World Health Organization (WHO). (2000). *General guidelines for methodologies on research and evaluation of traditional medicine.* http://apps.who.int/iris/bitstream/10665/66783/1/WHO_EDM_TRM_2000.1.pdf

World Health Organization (WHO). (2003). *WHO definition of health.* http://who.int/about/definition/en/print.html http://www.who.int/water_sanitation_health/bathing/srwe1/en/

World Health Organization (WHO). (2004). *Obesity: Prevention and managing the global epidemic.* Geneva. http://apps.who.int/iris/bitstream/10665/42330/1/WHO_TRS_894.pdf?ua=1

World Health Organization (WHO). (2013). *WHO traditional medicine strategy: 2014-2023.* http://apps.who.int/iris/bitstream/10665/92455/1/9789241506090_eng.pdf?ua=1

World Health Organization (WHO). (2014a). *Current edition of the WHO guidelines for drinking-water quality.* http://www.who.int/water_sanitation_health/dwq/guidelines2/en

World Health Organization (WHO). (2014b). *World Water Day.* http://www.who.int/pmnch/media/news/2014/water/en/

World Health Organization (WHO). (2014c). *Ten facts on obesity.* http://www.who.int/features/factfiles/obesity/en/

Worldwide Aquatic Bodywork Association (WABA). (2014). *Worldwide aquatic bodywork registry.* http://waba.forest.net:591/waba/FmPro?-db=wregistry&-lay=3search&-format=3search.htm&-error=3search.htm&-token.3=English&-token.9=xopenwater&openwater=1&-SortField=begindate&-max=25&-find

Wykle, M.O. (2003). Safety first. *Rehab Management, 16*(6), 24-27, 50.

Yoga Site. (2004). *Meditation.* http://www.yogasite.com/meditation.htm

Zhang, G.G., Bausell, B., Lao, L., Handwerger, B., & Berman, B.M. (2003). Assessing the consistency of traditional Chinese medical diagnosis: An integrative approach. *Alternative Therapies in Health and Medicine, 9*(1), 66-71.

INDEX

Page numbers followed by an italicized *f* indicate figures; and *t*, tables.

spa therapy, 55
special needs children, music therapy for, 72
specific gravity, 57
spinal manipulation, 4-5
spiritual healing, 115-120
    about, 12
    in African folk healing, 107-108
    types of, 117*t*
sprain treatments, African folk healers, 106
St. John's wort, uses/precautions, 10, 34, 39*t*, 41*t*
state regulations, nursing, 3
steam baths, 58
steam distillation, 24, 24*t*
steam inhalation, 27
stress reduction, 123-124, 126-127, 136-137
sun salutation, 84
Svadisthana chakra (yoga), 85
Swedish massage, 93, 94
swelling treatments, African folk healers, 106
symbolic healing rituals, 107-108
syncretic faith healing, 105, 107, 118
synthetics, 24*t*, 25

T
tai chi, 5
Taxol, 35*t*
tea shrub, 35*t*
tea tree, 23*t*, 25*t*
theophylline, 35*t*
Therapeutic Touch, 11, 91, 92, 93, 95-98
Therapeutic Touch Network of Ontario, 96
thyme, 23*t*, 25*t*
topical application of essential oils, 26
touch therapy, 91-99
    acupressure, 110
    Chinese massage, 111
    essential oils, 24
    reflexology, 45-52, 46*f*
    See also massage therapy
traditional healers, 10, 33-34, 105
Trager psychophysical integration, 4
transcendental meditation, 4
    See also meditation
turbulence, 57

U
Unitarian Energy Field, 97

V
vegetarian/vegan diets, 135
vinca major, hazards, 40*t*
Virginia Graeme Baker Pool & Spa Safety Act (P&SS Act), 63
Visuddha chakra (yoga), 85

vitamins, 4, 133-134
Vitamins and Minerals Amendment (1976), 35
voice-guided imagery, 75
volatility of essential oils, 20, 22, 26-27, 29

W
Warfarin, 41*t*
warm packs, 59
warm-up in yoga, 84
water temperature, aquatic therapy and, 63, 63*t*
water therapy, 55
water-borne infections, aquatic therapy and, 62
Watsu, 57, 59-60
weight loss diets, 134-135, 135*t*
whirlpool baths, 55
willow bark, 34, 35*t*
World Health Organization (WHO), 62, 116
wound-healing, African folk healers, 106
wraps, aquatic therapy as, 55, 59

Y
yama (yoga), 81, 82
yin and yang, 109, 109*f*, 110
ylang-ylang, 23*t*, 25*t*
yoga and meditation, 11, 79-88
Yoga Sutra (Patanjali), 80, 81
yohimbe, hazards, 40*t*, 41*t*

Z
Zen macrobiotics, 134
Zen Shiatsu, 57, 60
Zone Theory of Foot Reflexology, 47